BOOTCAMP360*

a complete fitness program

FOR BRIDES

The FEW, The PROUD, The FIT

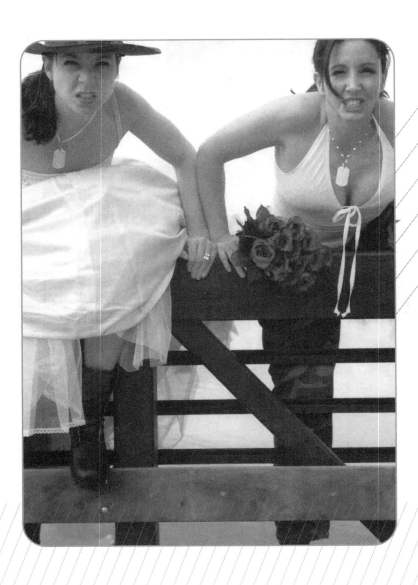

▲ HarperResource

An Imprint of HarperCollins*Publishers*

BOOTCAMP360

a complete fitness program

FOR BRIDES

The FEW, The PROUD, The FIT

The no-excuses, no-pain, no-gain plan of attack that
will get you fit for your wedding day and happily ever after

TAMARA KLEINBERG

HARPERCOLLINS BOOKS MAY BE PURCHASED FOR EDUCATIONAL, BUSINESS, OR SALES PROMOTIONAL USE. FOR INFORMATION, PLEASE WRITE: SPECIAL MARKETS DEPARTMENT, HARPERCOLLINS PUBLISHERS INC., 10 EAST 53RD STREET, NEW YORK, NY 10022.

ALL PHOTOGRAPHS AND TESTIMONIALS HAVE BEEN REPRINTED BY PERMISSION.

THIS BOOK IS WRITTEN AS A SOURCE OF INFORMATION ONLY. THE INFORMATION CONTAINED IN THIS BOOK SHOULD BY NO MEANS BE CONSIDERED A SUBSTITUTE FOR THE ADVICE OF A QUALIFIED MEDICAL PROFESSIONAL, WHO SHOULD ALWAYS BE CONSULTED BEFORE BEGINNING ANY NEW DIET, EXERCISE, OR OTHER HEALTH PROGRAM.

ALL EFFORTS HAVE BEEN MADE TO ENSURE THE ACCURACY OF THE INFORMATION CONTAINED IN THIS BOOK AS OF THE DATE PUBLISHED. THE AUTHOR AND THE PUBLISHER EXPRESSLY DISCLAIM RESPONSIBILITY FOR ANY ADVERSE EFFECTS ARISING FROM THE USE OR APPLICATION OF THE INFORMATION CONTAINED HEREIN.

FIRST EDITION

DESIGNED BY PLATINUM DESIGN, INC.

LIBRARY OF CONGRESS CATALOGING-IN-PUBLICATION DATA

KLEINBERG, TAMARA.
    BOOTCAMP360: A COMPLETE FITNESS PROGRAM FOR BRIDES: THE FEW, THE PROUD, THE FIT / TAMARA KLEINBERG.
      P. CM.
    INCLUDES INDEX.
    ISBN 0-06-072222-3
    1. PHYSICAL FITNESS FOR WOMEN. 2. BRIDES—HEALTH AND HYGIENE. 3. WEIGHT LOSS. I. TITLE.

RA778.K7125 2005
613'.04244—DC22

2004054367

05 06 07 08 09 WBC/RRD 10 9 8 7 6 5 4 3 2 1

ACKNOWLEDGMENTS

A heartfelt thank-you to my patient and loving husband, Mike, who has given me all the encouragement and confidence in the world. His romantic, creative marriage proposal and a simple "Will you marry me?" turned into the Bootcamp360 journey. He is the rock that keeps me sane. A special thank-you to my good friend and crutch, Tonya Bruno. Her support and help have been an essential part of Bootcamp360's success and my life. Marc and Kathy, thank you for believing in the idea and in me. Of course, none of this would have been possible without all the beautiful brides who have contributed to this book and the program. Last but not least, a big hug to Bootcamp360's first and toughest drill sergeant, Amy Holley. I have never met a woman with more energy and passion for helping women achieve their dreams. She is an integral part of Bootcamp360 and I hope always will be.

A special thank-you to the following people and places that contributed so generously to *Bootcamp360: A Complete Fitness Program for Brides.*

Peggy Irelan Photography
Real people, real moments
www.peggyirelan.com
Boulder and San Francisco

Amici Studios
Wedding Stylists
10 Fourth Street, Suite 103
Santa Rosa, California
(707) 575-9562

Outdoor Divas
Adventure clothing for women
www.outdoordivas.com
133 Pearl Street
Boulder, Colorado

Barbara Gehring
Actress, model, and comedian
www.barbaragehring.com

Trentadue Winery
www.trentadue.com
info@Trentadue.com
19170 Geyserville Avenue
Geyserville, California 95441-9603
(707) 433-3104/(888) 332-3032

Top Toque
Chef Dillon
chefdillon@yahoo.com

CONTENTS

ARE YOU READY TO BE ONE OF THE FEW, THE PROUD, THE FIT?

ANSWER THE FOLLOWING QUESTIONS AND FIND OUT IF YOU ARE READY TO BECOME A BOOTCAMP360 FOR BRIDES RECRUIT.

1. What are your three main weight-loss and fitness goals?

_____

_____

_____

2. How close to your three main weight-loss and fitness goals do you feel you are now?
   A. Nowhere near, I haven't started trying
   B. Not very close but I've started trying
   C. On the way but I have setbacks and plateaus
   D. Slowly getting there but I could use some help

3. When it comes to reaching your three main goals, where do you need the most support?
   A. In every aspect
   B. Getting motivated
   C. Staying on track
   D. Kicking it up a notch

4. How often do you exercise a week?
   A. Never
   B. Here and there but not consistently
   C. Usually 2–3 times a week
   D. 5–6 days a week or more

5. Overall, how consistent are your workouts?
   A. Not at all
   B. Every week is different
   C. Consistent but my workouts are no longer challenging
   D. I work out regularly but I am just going through the motions

6. How many days a week do you maintain a healthy diet?
   A. Never
   B. I get a healthy meal in once or twice a week
   C. I try regularly, but I am not consistent
   D. I eat a healthy and balanced diet regularly

7. How would you rate your motivation to reach your goals?
   A. I need some help even getting motivated
   B. It all depends on my mood
   C. I am usually motivated but I have bad days
   D. I have tons of motivation but I am still not reaching my goals

Mostly A's: Move Out, Soldier! It's time to get off that couch and start moving. No more procrastinating or putting it off until next week. For the first time you are going to discover what it truly takes to lose weight and tone up—and love every step of the way. The Bootcamp360 regime will walk you through the basics and be your trusted guide as you achieve your goals.

Mostly B's: Stay on Track! Time to get off that weight-loss roller coaster for good. You know what you need to do and now you are going to do it. It will be easier than ever to stay the course and achieve your dreams. Keep your eye on the prize, soldier, and the results will come.

Mostly C's: Kick It into Gear! You have what it takes but plateaus and setbacks are constantly getting in the way of your goals. Feelings of frustration seem to set you back even further. Never fear, Bootcamp360 will give you that extra shove you need to get the results you want. Plateaus and setbacks are a thing of the past with this challenging and fun regime.

Mostly D's: I Dare You! You know what it takes and aren't afraid of a little sweat, yet those goals still elude you. You are always searching for a new challenge, and have I got one for you! Stop going through the motions and step up to the Bootcamp360 regime—

finally make those goals a reality. As you are no stranger to hard work and dedication, this is the perfect program for you.

TAKE A MOMENT, SIT DOWN, AND ANSWER THESE QUESTIONS HONESTLY:

1. HAVE YOU GAINED FIVE POUNDS OR MORE SINCE YOU MET YOUR FIANCÉ?

2. IS THE PERSON LOOKING BACK AT YOU IN THE MIRROR LARGER THAN YOU THOUGHT SHE WAS?

3. IS THE DRESS OF YOUR DREAMS SLEEVELESS? STRAPLESS? OR EVEN BACKLESS?

4. DID WEDDING-DRESS SHOPPING LEAVE YOU DISAPPOINTED AND FRUSTRATED?

5. ARE YOU SERIOUSLY CONSIDERING TUMMY TUCKERS UNDER YOUR WEDDING DRESS?

6. DO YOU PLAN ON WEARING A LONG VEIL TO HIDE YOUR BACKSIDE?

7. IS YOUR FIRST FITTING QUICKLY APPROACHING AND YOU HAVEN'T HAD A CHANCE TO LOSE ALL THE WEIGHT YOU PROMISED YOURSELF YOU WOULD?

8. ARE YOU WORRIED THAT YOUR WEDDING PHOTOS WILL TURN INTO YOUR "BEFORE" PHOTOS?

9. DOES YOUR HONEYMOON INCLUDE A BEACH AND A BIKINI?

10. IS IT FINALLY TIME TO GET BACK INTO THE SHAPE YOU ONCE WERE?

IF YOU ANSWERED YES TO ANY OF THESE QUESTIONS, THEN YOU NEED TO TURN THIS PAGE AND START MOVING! NOT TOMORROW, NOT NEXT MONDAY . . . RIGHT NOW!

BOOTCAMP360★

a complete fitness program
FOR BRIDES

The FEW, The PROUD, The FIT

/

THE ORIGINAL RECRUIT

TAMARA GHANDOUR KLEINBERG
178 pounds
POUNDS LOST: 30
DRESS SIZES LOST: 4
BODY FAT % LOST: 7

There I was standing in front of the mirror, baffled. Why didn't my bra fit? Why did my favorite jeans make my love handles hang over my belt line? That couldn't possibly be me in the mirror. Was there something wrong with the mirror? Did my dryer shrink my clothes? Did I really gain that much weight?

As I stared into the mirror, I knew in my heart that I really had gained the weight, but I wasn't ready to admit it. Sure, sitting here today, I realize that my weight gain didn't happen overnight, but when that 178-pound woman was staring back at me, I couldn't face the truth. I didn't want to.

How did I let this happen? I could give you a million and one excuses to justify it, but I won't. In fact, excuses were my standard MO for quite some time. Instead, I will tell you the truth. Throughout my life, my weight had stayed relatively constant; to be honest, it was easy for me to be thin. I used to be fit and had an arsenal of exercises and sports that I enjoyed. In fact, I made it a priority to go to the gym a few times a week, run in the park with friends, play touch football on the weekends for fun, and even make fruit shakes for breakfast. To top if off, I walked to work and back almost every day. But in February of 2000 I moved to a new city with my boyfriend, bought a big SUV, and discovered fast food.

My lifestyle changed drastically with that move. I would go through the drive-through just to get coffee. I would drive to the gym, stop before I broke into a sweat on the treadmill, then drive to

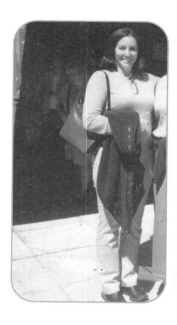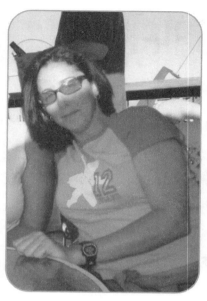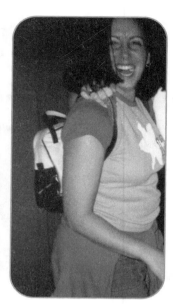

work, where I sat on my butt all day. After work, convinced that I was too tired to work out, I would sit in front of the TV for the night and snack away. My meal portions got larger in an attempt to match my boyfriend's portions.

Over eight months, I gained more than thirty pounds. It's not that I didn't see what was happening to me; it's that I chose to deny it. If someone had asked me back then if I was active, I would immediately have answered yes, without hesitation. But I knew deep down that wasn't true.

It was easy for me to deny that I had lost control. I had subconsciously chosen not to keep up those healthy habits and had elected to replace them with rationalizations and complacency. Ultimately I had selected to be fat instead of fit. Sound familiar? If I had chosen to see it, I would have been forced to make drastic changes. I honestly thought it was easier to be fat than it was to be fit.

By the start of 2001—weighing the most I had ever weighed at 178 pounds—I was resigned to being an unfit, fat girl. I blamed it on everything but myself: genetics, suburban life, age. You name it and I blamed it. I was resigned to a life of buying clothes from the back of the rack where they keep the big-girl sizes. I worked hard to make sure that before somebody took a photo of me, I had a chance to cover my stomach. (As you can see in one of the photos, I always had a purse or a sweater in front of my belly.) I would wear layer upon layer in the hope that it would cover up my thighs and butt. I actually have few photos from that time in my life; I truly hated getting in front of the camera. Perhaps if you take a look at your photo albums, you will find the same thing.

What was the breaking point? Ironically, it happened after one of the happiest days of my life. My boyfriend, bless his soul, created an elaborate surprise for his marriage proposal. It was romantic, surprising (although I did get my nails done just in case), and fun. He proposed in front of the house where we'd first met in California, seven years earlier. We spent the next day tasting wine and taking photos in the vineyards. Once again, I was all covered up. From the double chin down, I didn't want anyone to see me.

I returned home on cloud nine. All my friends were excited and we spent hours at lunch discussing my dream dress and the perfect place to hold the wedding. Weight forgotten, I felt that I would be the most beautiful bride ever and that this feeling would last forever. It did last . . . that is of course until I went dress shopping.

My girlfriends and I planned to go from shop to shop trying on all the dress styles, hoping to find the dress that would make me look as beautiful as any bride could look. I set out that morning with high hopes of finding the perfect dress.

But that never happened. I couldn't fit into *any* of the dresses. My thighs were too big, my back was too large, and my hips were certainly too wide. The salesclerk would stand behind me holding the dress up, since it wouldn't zip up past my lower back. After hours of torture, I went home and cried. I was not going to be the beautiful blushing bride I had envisioned for years. I went to bed that night feeling utterly destroyed. I had nightmares about my big fat body. The idea of walking down the aisle was no longer exciting or even appealing—it was a living nightmare!

The next morning I woke up feeling frustrated and depressed, turning to my usual routine of making coffee and breakfast. As I was putting cream in my coffee and butter on my toast, I realized that *I* could change how I looked and felt. *I* could become that beautiful, radiant bride who was hiding inside. *I* was solely responsible for changing my lifestyle. At that moment, I knew that my routine, my habits, and my complacency had to change.

Bootcamp360 was born on that fateful morning. I sat down and thought about all my past attempts to lose weight. All the fad diets, personal trainers, and programs I had tried and failed at miserably. I had counted calories, separated out food groups, restricted my carbohydrate intake, subscribed to online diets and exercise programs, and spent money on new clothing, trainers, and equipment I would never use. All of the books bought, e-mails received, and equipment purchased were now collecting dust and I was still my unfit, frustrated self.

Why did all those attempts fail? Even when I did lose weight, I easily gained it back the minute I went off the diet. Reviewing past attempts, I noticed a few common mistakes that I vowed not to make again. I vowed not to go on one of those diets that required a complete lifestyle makeover, since I could not sustain the plan for more than two weeks at a time. I would go to the grocery store and easily pay over $300 for a week's worth of food and spend hours making my meals for the next day. Forget it! It's much easier to order Chinese. Other diets didn't work because there was no sense of accountability. If I cheated, it didn't really matter because no one was around to see it. I considered them empty calories—after all, if no one is there to see me eat them, they can't really count, right? No one noticed if I didn't go to the gym. The truth is that deep down I knew what to do; I just wasn't doing it.

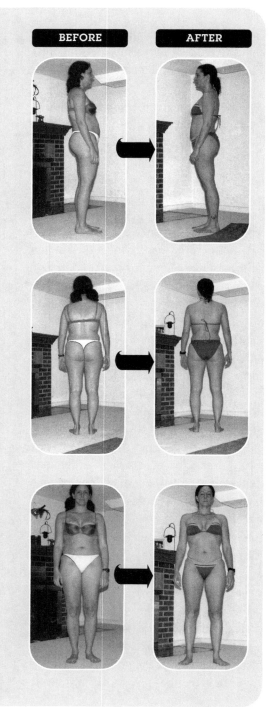

BEFORE	AFTER

This time I was going to do it my way, with a plan that combined common sense and personal tough love. I used my education and experience—both the motivational and accountability tools I'd learned through my BA in psychology and the discipline and structure I'd learned when training for my black belts in tae kwon do and kickboxing—and created a program that would work. In the pursuit of even more knowledge I obtained a national certification in personal training and weight management from the American Council of Exercise, as well as building my arsenal with courses in exercise physiology, anatomy, and kinesiology. I called my program Bridal Bootcamp.

I began with the four main staples of the Bootcamp program: Motivation, Accountability, Exercise, and Nutrition. At this point, I had all the motivation I needed. After all, I had the vision of the blushing bride pulsating through my head hourly. My next step was to put that motivation to good use and to set goals for myself to keep myself accountable. I weighed myself, took measurements, and measured my body-fat percentage as benchmarks so that I could calculate my progress. I even took photos so that I could objectively see the weight melting off my body. I then developed a comprehensive exercise and nutrition program, knowing that these were important to sustaining my weight goal.

From the beginning and most important, I began taking responsibility for and careful account of my actions. I no longer allowed myself to succumb to my old, unhealthy habits. Month after month the results became an even greater inspiration and motivation. I watched as the extra weight, inches, and fat melted off my body. Every month I set a goal of losing five pounds, and in six months I had lost all the excess weight and dropped 7 percent body fat.

The photos I took of myself proved I was trimming down and toning up. My love handles and excess fat disappeared and were replaced with the hourglass figure I had once had. I began to exude confidence and felt happy again. My energy soared. I was back in the game and engaged in life (not just to my fiancé). More important, my dress was no longer my only motivation; the feeling of being fit and energized became my second "drill sergeant." I continued to feel strong and vital beyond just a week or two, and I realized that the end goal was not my wedding day but to feel this way forever.

Friends and family were dazzled as the pounds kept melting away. "How did you do it?" they kept asking. When I told them of my bootcamp program, they wanted in on all of its secrets. In fact, one day before my wedding, a family friend called and asked me if she could also do it. She wanted to lose some weight and tone up for her own wedding and had heard through the grapevine about my results. It was then that I realized that I had something that could truly help others just as I'd helped myself. At that moment, Danielle in Toronto officially became the second bride recruit. I set pen to paper and put Bridal Bootcamp into a workbook. For about six months she followed my instructions, stayed the course, and successfully graduated from Bootcamp recruit to the Reserves (the portion of the program where you maintain your success). Her success made me believe that this program would work for brides everywhere.

So in September of 2002, after I returned from our honeymoon, I rented an aerobics room inside a spa and opened the doors for business. As word spread, more and more brides enlisted in our thirteen-week basic training. Soon TV, newspapers, magazines, and radio were calling me for interviews and stories. Our enlistment grew every month until we eventually grew beyond our little studio.

Since the inception of the organization, we have grown: we now have bootcamps for anyone who wants to get fit, including new moms' and special corporate programs, and we also keep our old recruits in line with Reserves bootcamp. While bootcamp for brides will always be at the heart of the business, I am thrilled to offer the bootcamp philosophy of tough love and common sense to women of all walks of life. Our flagship studio sits in one of the fittest cities in the country—Denver, Colorado—and it enlists from across the country and in Canada. While I maintain the title of Founder and Original Recruit, the newly titled Bootcamp360 organization now has many talented and tough drill sergeants who help recruits of all shapes and sizes find their inner "athlete."

While my experience has driven the vision of the business, it is the input of hundreds of brides that truly makes this program work. I made it a point to get their feedback every step of the way, asking them what worked, what didn't, and what tips they had based on their experience. They have helped this program evolve into what it is today. While I have been doing this for a while now, I still find that it is the recruits who have the best tips and tricks. Each person is unique and finds innovative ways to cut out foods, get motivated to work out, and stay on course. These tips and tricks are sprinkled throughout the book so that you can also benefit from their valuable input.

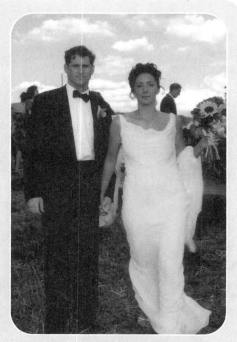

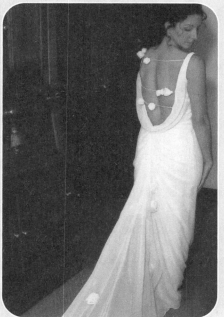

Tamara and Michael Kleinberg on the day she'd been preparing for.

Take advantage of not just my experience and expertise, but also of the experience of hundreds of brides. This book is the culmination of all the above, and it is your drill sergeant and resource book for your wedding and for your life. Everything that you learn in this book can be applied long after you get married.

My eyes are wide open now; I know that it is easier to be fit than to be fat. Hopefully *Bootcamp360: A Complete Fitness Program for Brides* will teach you that same lesson that began for me over four years ago.

Now, read on, soldier, and begin marching with the hundreds of brides around the country who have walked confidently down the aisle and into their new lives.

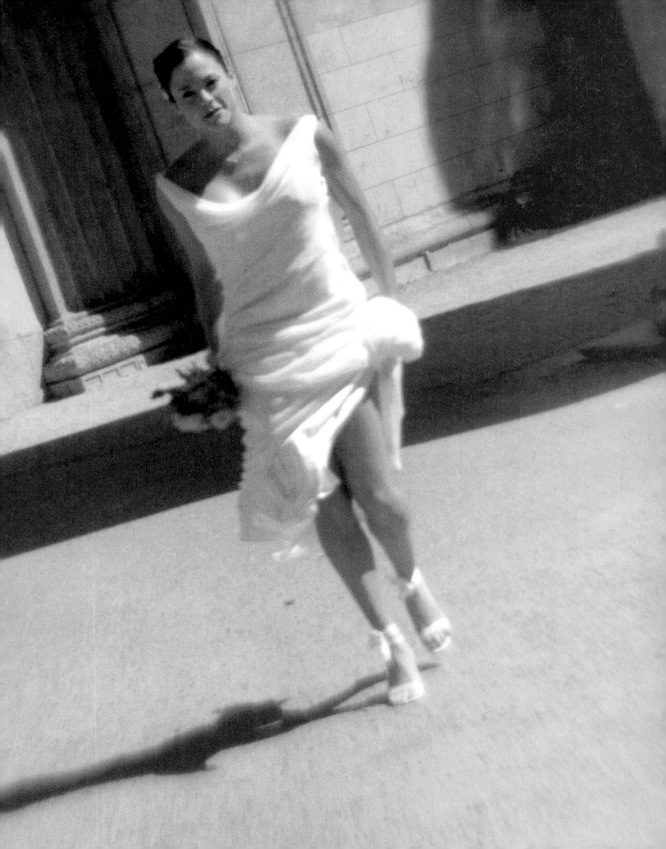

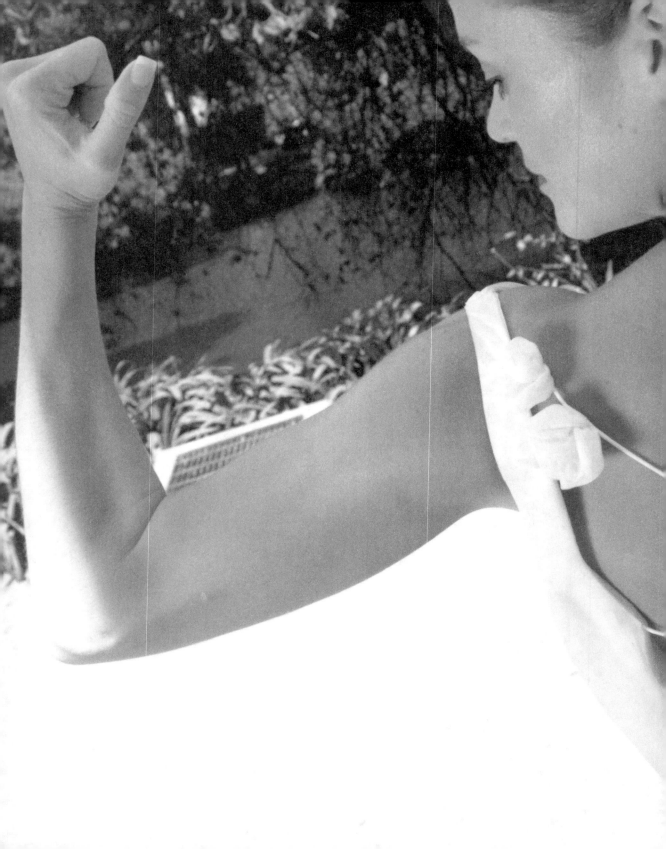

A WEDDING PLANNER FOR YOUR BODY

PLANNING CHECKLIST

Are you ready? As you read this chapter, go over our checklist to make sure you have done every-thing you need to do to start transforming your body. This step-by-step checklist has been grouped according to the four major components of the Bootcamp360 program (Motivation, Accountability, Exercise, and Nutrition) so that you can easily begin marching toward success. And unlike your wedding checklist, where you are concerned with how many of your parents' friends need to be in-vited, this checklist is all about you—and only you.

MOTIVATION AND COMMITMENT

Commitment Contract signed

ACCOUNTABILITY

Benchmark
- ❑ Cloth tape measure
- ❑ Weight scale

Weight _____

Inches

Arm _____

Bust _____

Waist_____

Hips _____

Thigh _____

Clothing size _____

Set your overall goals _____
_____
_____

Set your monthly goals _____
_____
_____

Make photocopies of your Report-In log (page 31)

EXERCISE

- ❑ Buy all your Bootcamp360 gear:

  Resistance band; Jump rope; Exercise ball; good workout outfit. Three sets
  of free weights; Make photocopies of exercise logs (pages 232–245)

NUTRITION

Make photocopies of your Plan and Progress logs (pages 226–228).

Congratulations, you are now armed with all the tools you need to begin the Bootcamp360 regime. I wish you the best of luck in your efforts and look forward to seeing the results on your wedding day.

Think of this book as the wedding planner for your body. You are about to invest in the most perfect and expensive dress you will ever wear. You aren't going to spend all that money and attention to detail on your dress and leave your body to chance.

Photographers and videographers will be capturing you from every angle, especially during those special moments when you aren't paying attention. They won't prompt you to stand up straight or suck in your stomach, so you need to be in shape and guarantee that every shot they take from every angle captures how truly fabulous you look. It may only be one day, but the photos, video, and new healthy lifestyle will last a lifetime.

Whether your wedding is a year, six months, or three weeks away, now is the time to take action. It's never too early or too late to sculpt a gun-ready physique.

Plus, the Bootcamp360 regime will not only give you the body you want, but will also help relieve the stress and pressure of planning a wedding. You know what I'm talking about: stress is what you feel when your future mother-in-law calls you to add a few people to your guest list whom you've never even met. It is that fight-or-flight feeling that overcomes you when your florist tells you that the flowers you wanted are out of season. It is the unbearable frustration and anx-

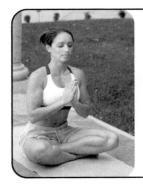

Real Brides: Tips from the Trenches

To alleviate that heart-pounding fight-or-flight feeling, make a ten-minute appointment with yourself daily to do some body and mind relaxation exercises. Yoga, meditation, deep breathing, and aromatherapy will instantly relax your spirit and allow you to reenter the wedding world calm and motivated.

iety you experience while trying to balance work and planning a wedding. It's perfectly natural to feel that you are being pulled in every direction and even overwhelmed by the monumental task at hand.

But listen up, soldier! A doughnut and a TV show do not relieve stress; exercise and eating healthy do. Our bodies are like pressure cookers, and we need outlets for all that bottled-up stress. Exercise is the best way to relieve that stress. Feeling extra-annoyed? Take a kickboxing class to get out some of that aggression. Just received that dreaded phone call from the dress shop saying your dress is going to be three weeks late? Go for a hard jog. So the next time you are feeling the crunch, get out there and sweat . . . and that's a direct command from me to you. Better yet, it is a command you give yourself. Most important, promise yourself that you will find the time to do it all—and love it. Bootcamp360 will help minimize your stress while making you into the beautiful blushing bride.

Real Brides: Tips from the Trenches

You don't need green taffeta bridesmaid dresses to make you look fabulous. Garish and fluffy bridesmaids' dresses are visual distractions to the centerpiece—the bride.

To be the perfect centerpiece, remember that every dress is as unique as the bride who wears it. Each figure has the perfect fit. Follow these guidelines as you try on wedding dresses:

Full Figure (round hips and butt, a bit of a belly, full breasts) . . . A classic ball-gown style (trim upper body with a full bodice) will hide quite a bit. A corset-style top with a more structured ribbing will bring in the waistline, giving you the appearance of a slim upper body.

Apple-Shape Figure (heavy in the midsection) . . . An Empire waist (high waistline typically directly under the chest, falling into a slimmer skirt) will deemphasize your midsection, giving you a leaner look.

Hourglass Figure (curves in all the right places) . . . An A-line or princess-style dress (hallmarks of this dress are the vertical seams that seamlessly flow from the shoulders to a flared skirt) is a slimming shape for a womanly body, hiding the flaws and highlighting your assets.

Pear-Shape Figure (trim on top, heavy on the bottom) . . . A traditional ball gown (trim on top with a full, rounded skirt) is the key to hiding the lower body by drawing attention to your sleek shoulders and neck. A strapless or spaghetti-strap style will further emphasize your trim top.

Slim Figure (less curves, more of a straight-line body) . . . Showcase the slinky mermaid style (body-hugging dress with a sunshine-flared bottom) to bring out curves you didn't even know you had.

While your weight will change and your body will tone, your body type and figure will remain the same.

Spend time looking for that perfect dress—the one that instantly makes your feel like a bride. Try every style, cut, and fabric until you known you've found the one.

If you're asking yourself how to look your best in your dress and adopt a healthy lifestyle, Bootcamp360 has the answers you need: it can't help you choose your dress, caterer, or china pattern, but it can help you look fantastic for your wedding and for the rest of your life.

In keeping with the idea of getting married, Bootcamp360 for Brides promotes lifestyle changes. You just made a major lifestyle change yourself—single girl to girlfriend to now fiancée. Bootcamp360 will be your trusted drill sergeant as you transition from fiancée to wife. All too often, brides wait until a few weeks before their wedding before realizing that they don't look how they want. They end up resorting to fad diets and pills that inevitably don't work. When they don't lose the weight, they end up looking unhealthy and unhappy on their wedding day.

The truth is that quick fixes and fad diets don't work. Any diet that promises immediate and drastic results is only fooling you. You may lose ten pounds in one week, but I guarantee you will gain it back in the second week. Do you want to gain the weight back on your honeymoon? Of course not! If you are losing more than one to two pounds a week, you are not only losing fat but valuable water and muscle mass as well. This is not healthy for you in the short term or in the long run. You may see a smaller number on the scale, but you will also feel lethargic and tired. There is no miracle pill, diet, or way to avoid exercise when it comes to weight loss and toning up. It's about action and results!

Many diets and plans out there focus only on your diet or on your exercise. It doesn't make sense to focus only on exercise or only on your diet. If you succeed in one element of fitness and fail in another, you will never see any results. It will feel as if you are constantly running in place. You can't exercise and then eat everything at the buffet table. Conversely, dieting without exercise can lead to a loss of muscle mass as well as fat, giving you an unhealthy, almost sickly look. You want to look amazing on your big day, not emaciated.

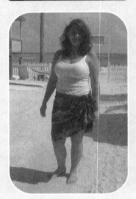 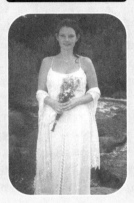
Bootcamp360 for Brides returns to methods that are tried-and-true to deliver results that will last long past the honeymoon, not just a week or a month. After all, you want to be his better half, not his better three-quarters! Fad diets actually want you to fail so you will return over and over. Bootcamp360 was developed to be the exact opposite. It was developed for a lasting lifestyle change, using your wedding as a positive and motivating catalyst. You certainly don't want to lose weight only to gain it all back within weeks of your wedding! I know you want your weight loss ef-

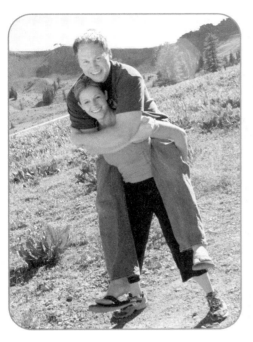

forts to be successful now and forever—just like your marriage.

There are a few mantras to live by if you want to lose weight and get fit. First and foremost, you must make exercise a priority. The more you exercise, the more calories you burn. In many ways, losing weight and gaining muscle is a mathematical equation. If you are eating more than you are expending, you will undoubtedly gain weight. Your body will store the excess energy as fat. You need to create a deficit by expending more calories than you take in, and the best and most effective way to do this is regular exercise. You certainly expend some energy while at rest, but your energy expenditure increases dramatically when you begin to move. For example, on average, walking expends six calories per minute, jogging ten calories, and running fifteen to twenty.

Research has shown time and time again that you need a balance of aerobic activity, strength, and flexibility for optimal health. This balance creates a better body. Second, food is a source of fuel for the body and must be treated as such. Stop picking up the fork or opening the fridge when you aren't hungry. Stop eating high-calorie, low-nutrient foods such as pasta, chips, and sweets. Tip the scale in the exact opposite direction. Eat foods that are high in nutrients and low in calories that will give you energy and stamina. Mother Nature makes certain foods for a reason—the human body needs them. Vegetables, fruits, grains, and legumes are excellent

Real Brides: Tips from the Trenches

Buy, then try. We've all heard the horror stories about brides who bought their wedding dress two sizes too small but never trimmed down and ended up looking like a stuffed sausage in it. A good bridal shop will insist that you buy your wedding dress at your current size, not your intended size. Usually there is a three- to four-month wait, unless you buy off the rack, before your dress arrives for your first fitting. This is usually a few months prior to your wedding date. Our advice: buy your dress and then trim down. This will give you enough time to lose the weight, tone up the body, and make a much-needed appointment for alterations.

examples and should constitute the majority of your diet. Eat less, exercise more . . . and that's an order!

In Bootcamp360 it's all about common sense and methods that have been proven time and time again. You will achieve long-term results through short-term goals.

I truly believe that every woman has the "hot" bride inside; she just needs to find a way to unleash her. If you do the work and follow the program, she will emerge. You will see her in the photos, on the scale, in your clothes, and—most important—smiling back at you in the mirror as you prepare to walk down the aisle.

BOOTCAMP360 OVERVIEW

Bootcamp360 training is much more than just push-ups and floral bouquets. It's time to discover your inner strength and to learn valuable skills that will always be with you.

If this is the first time you are attempting to stick to a fitness program, stand front and center—you can do this. Remember to take it day by day. Every step forward is a step in the right direction. Start at your level. This is about doing your best, not the best of the person lapping you around the park. They too once started in the same place you are today. Just remember that if you stick with the

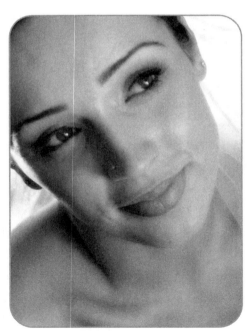

program, someday you will be the person lapping ahead of other runners. The drill sergeants and your fellow recruits who have contributed to this book are always there for you, holding you accountable for your actions and supporting you when you need to renew your inspiration for accepting the Bootcamp360 challenge.

To stick to your program you need to hold yourself accountable and keep your motivation strong. This is why you, as a bride-to-be, will do it all . . . Motivation, Accountability, Exercise, and Nutrition. You've dreamed of this moment your whole life—don't shortchange yourself now!

Leave your excuses at the door!

The above motto is posted on the door of my Denver studio as a reminder to recruits that when entering the bootcamp program, they need to expect nothing but the best from themselves. Even though you will not be physically walking through the door, you need to mentally envision yourself marching into my studio and turning into a healthier, happier you.

The following exercise has helped hundreds of recruits do just that. Consider it the doorway into your own bootcamp studio. This exercise will break you down and then build you back up again—just like bootcamp.

Perception is reality. From here on out we are going to turn on the positive perception and let that drive our decision-making process. Take a moment to write down all the negative excuses you allow yourself to use.

- **"I didn't exercise today because [fill in the blank]."**
- **"I drank a pot of coffee this morning because [fill in the blank]."**
- **And my favorite: "I'll start tomorrow, not today, because [fill in the blank]."**

It is important that you be honest and truthful with yourself. If being lazy is your basic excuse, write it down. If you think you are always too busy, write that down too.

EXCUSES

Once you have fully completed the excuses box with all your excuses, put a big X over it. You no longer own these excuses and can therefore no longer use them. I don't want to hear any of these come out of your mouth. They are out of your head, on this paper, and never to be used again.

Let's start fresh. Take a deep breath and clear your mind. Think about all the positive reasons you have for being healthy.

- **"I exercise because [fill in the blank]."**
- **"I had a salad for lunch because [fill in the blank]."**
- **"I turned down martini happy hour because [fill in the blank]."**

Again, be honest. Your reasons can range from "because I look hot" to "because I have more confidence."

Now take a look at the reasons box containing all the positive reasons. These are your new excuses and you can use them anytime. Stay motivated, stay strong, and think about how you feel when you do the right thing.

Bootcamp360 basic training is composed equally of the following four pillars: Motivation, Accountability, Exercise, and Nutrition. Consider all of them to be the wheels on your car. If you don't have even one of them, the car will not drive. Although these pillars are placed in a specific order to make the start of your program easy, they are all necessary components of your success.

Real Brides: Tips from the Trenches

My goal was to lose twenty pounds. My wedding dress sat in my closet until I reached my goal. I desperately wanted to try it on and get it fitted, but I waited until I lost the weight. It was the best thing I ever did. I looked so good when I finally tried it on I couldn't believe it!
—*Recruit Jenny*

GEARING UP: MOTIVATION

This is the first component for a good reason—without motivation, the other three components are meaningless. The way I measure the motivation of potential clients is by the initial conversation we have. I can always place the person in one of three categories. About 20 percent of the potential recruits I talk to don't even need convincing; they just say, "Sign me up!" The next 60 percent have the motivation but may have other concerns that we work out in a few conversations before ultimately the majority of them join. The last 20 percent have no motivation or intention of joining Bootcamp360; they just want an excuse to continue with their unhealthy lifestyle. They never enlist.

You have to ask yourself which category you fall into. If you are part of the first two, great! This is the program for you. If you are part of that last 20 percent, this is not for you and you need to put this book down and walk away. Remember, this is bootcamp, a program designed for the motivated and dedicated.

Okay, good. That you are reading on proves that you are a tried-and-true soldier, ready to con-

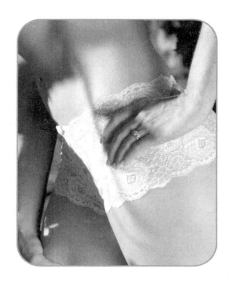

quer the rigors of training and full of the motivation it takes. Remember, every day is an opportunity to make your big day perfect. When you think of it that way, why wouldn't you exercise and eat well? Staying motivated, however, is really about getting through the obstacle course of life and, right now, wedding planning. We will maneuver through life and turn every day from here on out into a healthy one.

Experience tells us that lack of focus is the main reason most of us fail at our fitness and weight-loss efforts. How often have you sat on the couch watching TV for hours instead of getting up and exercising? Motivation can fluctuate monthly, weekly, or even daily. However, you are only getting married once, so you need to make sure every moment counts. You can't afford to let your motivation wane for a month or even a couple of days at a time. Whether you have one year, seven months, or just three months to plan your wedding and trim your body, your motivation will dictate how well you do. As a Bootcamp360 recruit you will start with lots of motivation and gain even more through momentum and focus.

Hup to and say "I do" to these motivational tools that will keep you focused and on course. The goal here is to implement motivational tools that will keep your energy high. And you will need a lot of it as you get closer to your wedding weekend.

"I Do's" of Motivation

I Do #1: Visualization
I Do #2: Rewards
I Do #3: Questions
I Do #4: Adventure
I Do #5: Training

I DO #1: VISUALIZATION   You probably spend a lot of time visualizing the details of your wedding: the bouquets, the candles on the table, and the music that plays as your guests sit down to their dinner. Include the new, fit, and trim you in those visualizations. Your new visualized self-image will drive your success.

Visualize the new you as you go to sleep at night. Cut out photos of your wedding dress and put a photo of your head on it. You can do the same with inspirational photos from fitness magazines.

I DO #2: REWARDS   Set monthly, weekly, and even daily rewards. It is healthy and motivating to reward yourself for big accomplishments like reaching your monthly goals, or small accomplishments like getting an extra workout in even though you are feeling tired and overwhelmed. Full-body massages, facials, pedicures, and relaxation time make magnificent rewards.

Real Brides: Tips from the Trenches

Keep a photo of your wedding dress on your bathroom mirror or inside your closet so that you can start every day with a smile on your face and with your goals in mind. Don't want your finacé to see the dress? Keep a photo in your makeup drawer or in your wallet. Take a few minutes every day to look at your photo and think about the new body that is going to showcase your fabulous dress.

I DO #3: QUESTIONS   As you're driving home from work looking forward to plopping down on the couch for the night, ask yourself, "Do I want to go for a long walk with the dog or do I want to feel guilty tomorrow?" Does that cake taste better than it feels to be fit? No, ma'am, it doesn't. You will eventually find the right questions for every situation.

Clearly your wedding is the best motivator you have. Finishing every question with ". . . or do I want to look amazing in my wedding dress?" will get you the answer you need almost every time to make the right choices.

Real Brides: Tips from the Trenches

Get fit your wedding . . . and for your table settings. At our wedding, we gave each table the name of a place we had been rather than the traditional numbers. Each table was named after a park, trail, or trip we had taken and included a photo of us at that spot. We hiked, snowshoed, and traveled until we had all of our fifteen tables. It was a lot of fun and helped both of us stay fit and active. —*Recruit Cori*

I DO #4: ADVENTURE   This is the perfect time to get out there and try something new. Are there trails in your neighborhood that you have never explored? Is there a class at the gym that you have never tried?

I DO #5: TRAINING   Many recruits stay motivated by signing up for local charity walks, midnight bike rides, and 10K races. This often helps give brides short-term structure and focus during an often chaotic time. Keep in mind that you don't need to go for time, beat the triathlete standing next to you, or even run. It's about doing your best at your fitness level. Every race, walk, or ride includes everyone from seasoned athletes to first-time participants.

Real Brides: Tips from the Trenches

Worried about bra fat hanging over your strapless dress? Tone up your arms by adding "negative" push-ups to your daily routine. Get into push-up position either on your toes or on your knees. Start at the top position, farthest from the floor. Slowly lower yourself until you can't hold the position any longer. The object is to take as long as possible to lower your body to the floor. Don't worry about the second part of the push-up. Do at least four to five of these a night for magnificent arms and a toned back.

MAKE THE COMMITMENT   This is an important part of the program. It solidifies your desire to reach your goals and your dedication to yourself.

Say these phrases out loud in front of a mirror. Don't laugh. Once you see and hear yourself commit, you will hold yourself more accountable for your actions and will be more successful.

These are the vows you need to make to yourself.

As a recruit you will commit to the following:

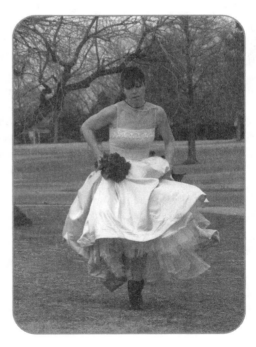

I will always give 100 percent.
I will take responsibility for my actions.
I will get the support and help I need.
I will have fun and enjoy the process.
I will reach my wedding day at my best.

Sign here to show that you agree to the above and are ready to become a recruit and start the Bootcamp360 for Brides regime:

Signed: _____

CONGRATULATIONS!   You are now officially a recruit. The countdown to your wedding and your new physique has begun. Check this off your list and move out, recruit . . . you have a wedding to plan and a body to shape!

BOOTCAMP360 SUCCESS STORY

RECRUIT JENNY

"I've seen all the pictures along with our wedding video, and I can honestly look at them and feel so good with how I looked that day."

BODY FAT % LOST: 3

SOMETHING OLD

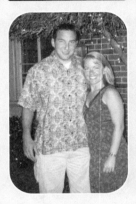

SOMETHING NEW

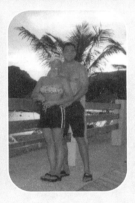

I never really felt fat, but I definitely didn't look like I was in shape. Some of the strapless dresses I tried on were cut in such a way that I would have this fold of skin squishing out from the sides, between my arm and armpit. *So* not pretty!

Before enlisting in bootcamp, I felt thick and squishy. I never considered myself fat, per se, but I had certainly lost the athletic look I had in college. I felt insecure about wearing certain outfits and definitely didn't feel attractive in a bathing suit. I was about to turn thirty and it hit me that my body definitely wasn't what it used to be. Brides-to-be are in a different place than regular people and they have special needs. I felt like these people might actually know what I was going through and could help me get to a place I was never before able to get to on my own.

I had never done a program that I stuck with long enough to actually see results. I began to wonder if it was even possible. But because it was so easy and motivating to stay with the Bootcamp360 program, I got results without even realizing it. I was having fun and losing weight—a combination you rarely experience. It was such a great feeling of accomplishment and motivated me to work even harder, knowing that I actually could make things happen. My confidence level increased and I started wearing cuter clothes again!

Other people noticed a difference in my shape and that's what made me feel good. I felt like my old self—my college self, the thin, active, athletic self. I felt more empowered because I realized that even though it can be tough and challenging, I actually can make a change.

On my wedding day I felt great! I felt confident . . . with not one bit of insecurity. I felt like I was glowing. For once, I had no reservations about all the photos being taken of me. I actually enjoyed it.

GEARING UP: ACCOUNTABILITY

Okay, now you are committed. With that comes taking responsibility for your own actions. Repeat after me, *I am going to take accountability for my actions!*

"I Do's" of Accountability

I Do #1: Benchmarking
I Do #2: Overall Goals
I Do #3: Monthly Goals
I Do #4: Logs
I Do #5: Wedding Party Battle Buddies

Accountability is a fundamental element of Bootcamp360. All too often we give in to unhealthy choices—or just plain laziness—without answering to anyone. It is time to change that.

Have a "take no prisoners" attitude in both your wedding planning and body sculpting. Accountability will keep you on track as you inch closer to your wedding day. First and foremost you must hold yourself accountable for your actions. Involving your fiancé, friends, and family—beyond going to bridal expos with you—will be a rich and rewarding experience for everyone.

I DO #1: BENCHMARKING A large part of accountability is benchmarking. Your benchmark is the point from which you start the program and a way to measure your progress at different points along the way. Your benchmark consists of your weight, your measurements, and your clothing size. As you go through this section, an example of a real bootcamp recruit's experience will be there to guide you every step of the way.

To determine your benchmark, you need the following items:

Cloth Tape Measure

Buy a cloth tape measure. It is easier and more accurate than using a plastic measure, which doesn't have any bend to it. Better yet, to make it easier, pick a trusted friend or family member to do your measurements; just make sure the same person does your measurements every month.

As you get ready for your dress fittings, you will want to make sure that you are toning up in all the right places: arms, bust, waist, hips, and thighs. I guarantee that going to your first, or last, dress fitting knowing that you have lost fifteen inches off your body will make you feel great. You will feel even better when they tell you that your wedding dress will have to be taken in by three sizes!

Weight Scale

If you don't have one already, go out and get a good scale. Having a scale at home also means that you can weigh in at the same time and on the same day. You will weigh in once a week as you work toward your monthly goals. It is extremely important that you weigh in only once a week: no more, no less. Your weight can fluctuate daily depending on what you ate, the time of day, etc. Weighing yourself every day will only drive you crazy.

Now that you have those two items, you are ready to benchmark your starting point.

EXAMPLE: REAL RECRUIT SARAH

Benchmarking

Before I could set my goals, I had to determine where I was currently. I benchmarked day one of my bootcamp regime. Think of it like your wedding budget. You can't go out and spend without knowing your limits. You can't determine your goals if you don't know your starting point. Losing twenty pounds is a perfectly reasonable goal if you are starting at a higher weight, but it isn't if you truly only have ten pounds to lose. In that case, you will want to consider not only weight but size as well.

To begin, I dusted off my bathroom scale and stepped on, measured myself (letting it all hang out), and put on a pair of jeans that really fit me. Here are my benchmarking results:

Date: November 15, 2002
Weight: 176 pounds
Inches:
    Arm: 13
    Bust: 39
    Waist: 31
    Hips: 42
    Thigh: 27
Clothing Size: 14 in jeans

Along with benchmarking my weight, measurements, and size, I took front, back, and side photos of my body every month. I did not like the dreaded photos at first, but I was incredibly proud as I watched the pounds melt away. At the end of the program, I laid the photos out on a table and could visibly see the fat disappear and the muscle appear.

Real Brides: Tips from the Trenches

Snap a photo. Not sure if your wedding dress hides the flaws and accentuates the assets? Before you head out to the bridal shops, load your camera with some film and stuff it into your purse. Every time you try on a dress you love, snap a photo. A few days later, after you've given your brain a chance to relax, lay all the photos on your coffee table. You will see the dresses in a whole new light. Put a large X over the wedding dresses that don't flatter your figure and a star on those that are still in the running.

YOUR TURN!

Benchmarking

With your dress in mind and a pen in your hand, let's begin by benchmarking where you are today. You must know where you start in order to know how successful you will be. You will benchmark all the angles of fitness: weight, inches across your body, and size. On page 31 you will find the chart you will use to benchmark, write down your goals, and report on your progress. Earmark the page; you will come back to it frequently. You will notice that the chart has enough columns for six months' worth of recruit reports. If you have enlisted in the program with more than six months to go before your wedding, simply photocopy the page so that you have enough columns to report your progress. If you have less time, simply begin reporting at the appropriate month.

Weighing Yourself

Go ahead and step on the scale. Again, make sure that you start with the same scale you intend to use throughout the program. Make a note of what you are wearing (if anything) and which shoes (if any), so that you can be consistent at each weigh-in. Don't be afraid of the scale. Just write the number down knowing that changes are close at hand.

Measuring Yourself

Measure yourself in five places: arm, bust, waist, hips, and thigh. The key to making this count is to do them in the same place each time. Follow these guidelines for making your measurements consistent. Use your body as a road map by designating freckles or birthmarks as measuring points.

Arm: On your right side, measure between the top of your shoulder and the pointy part of your elbow. At the halfway point, measure your arm circumference.

Bust: Measure around your chest at the nipple line.

Waist: Measure the circumference of your waist where your torso naturally indents, not where your pants fit.

Hips: Measure the circumference of your hips where you can feel the top of your hipbones. This is usually slightly below the belly-button line.

Thigh: On your right side, at the halfway point between the top of your hipbone and your kneecap, measure the circumference of your thigh.

Clothing size: Pull out a pair of jeans or any other nonstretchy clothing from your closet and try them on. If they fit, that is the size you should write down. If they are extremely tight, go up a size in clothing.

Step on the scale, measure yourself, pull out an outfit, and report back. Write the results of your benchmarking in the table below. Make sure you mark the date as well.

Recruit: _____'s Benchmark

Day One (Date): _____

Weight: _____

Inches:

       Arm: _____

       Bust: _____

       Waist: _____

       Hips: _____

       Thigh: _____

Clothing Size: _____

I DO #2: OVERALL GOALS   Now that you know your starting point, you can realistically determine your overall goals. Just think, when you decide to plan your wedding, what do you do? You begin by making the bigger decisions. You choose the type of wedding—outdoorsy, modern, traditional, or formal—as well as the date and place for your ceremony and reception. After deciding on the major issues (overall goals), the next step is to break down all the details of the wedding—all the little things (monthly goals) you need to do to get the job done. In the first month you must make appointments to preview the work of potential photographers and set up tastings with caterers. A month later you will sample music, decide on your photographer, and start shopping around for wedding dresses. This checklist continues on until all the elements of your wedding are in place. We are going to tackle your weight-loss and fitness goals the same way: one check mark at a time, one month at a time.

Real Recruit Sarah

Obviously, it would have been unrealistic and unhealthy for me to try to lose all that weight in one or two months. I would have gained it all back by the time I reached my wedding. I had to determine what a healthy weight loss is for someone like me. I'm five feet eight inches with a medium build. I decided to lose thirty pounds before my big day so I would look sexy in my wedding dress. This was a healthy and realistic goal given my height and starting weight. I then set my overall goals for the next six months. I thought about how much weight I wanted to lose, the clothes I wanted to wear, and how fit I truly wanted to be.

I wanted to make sure that I didn't just focus on my weight, so I added a fitness objective to balance out my goals. A fitness goal should be something that you can train for. For example, will you be hiking or kayaking on your honeymoon? Is there an upcoming event you would like to participate in? If you get winded after thirty minutes of aerobic exercise, being able to work out for sixty minutes without stopping is a great goal.

My overall goals were to lose thirty pounds, get back to a size 8, and run a 10K without walking.

I made these goals knowing that my most important short-term goal was to be beautiful and thin on my wedding day. My long-term goal was to change my life for the better.

YOUR TURN!

Determine Overall Goals

Now that you know your benchmark, it's time to determine a reasonable goal for yourself. Do you have any fitness goals you would like to accomplish? What would you like your weight to be as you slip into your wedding dress? Would you like to sport a sexy bikini on the beach? Go ahead and fill out the statement below.

My overall goals are to _____, _____, and _____.

I DO #3: MONTHLY GOALS

Real Recruit Sarah

Thinking about losing thirty pounds, three dress sizes, and running a 10K was totally overwhelming. Breaking it down into small tasks made it possible. Thinking about losing five to seven pounds a month, one dress size, and running a few extra miles a week were attainable tasks that I could touch and feel. Knowing that weight loss of one to two pounds a week is healthy, I set my monthly goals.

Every month I would set new goals and take the necessary steps to achieve them. At the end of every four weeks I would go back, chart my progress, and set new goals for the next month.

After only six months of the bootcamp program, I lost thirty pounds, was back into a size 8, ran a 10K without stopping, and decreased my body fat from 28 to 21 percent. (The healthy range for adult women is 21 to 25 percent body fat.) My dress arrived six months after I started the program—it was three sizes too big for me and ready to go to the tailor's.

Real Brides: Tips from the Trenches

Have your teeth whitened a few weeks before your wedding. But once you do, refrain from red wine, coffee, tea, and soda. It will help your smile stay white and your skin stay bright.

YOUR TURN!

Reaching Your Monthly Goals

Your monthly goals are important and we want to make sure you are headed down the right path. You don't want to wait three weeks to find out that you haven't made as much progress as you would have liked. To avoid this, check your progress weekly: no more, no less. Use the weekly progress report in "Bootcamp360 Resources" at the end of this book. Continually photocopy that page and use it weekly.

Weighing in can be one of the best indicators of your progress. Weigh in once a week only, on the same scale, same time, and same day. Weighing in any more than once a week will absolutely drive you crazy. As women, we tend to lend too much weight (pun intended) to the number on the scale. This is why you will also measure your body, take photos, and set fitness goals.

I DO #4: LOGS   Using the monthly "Report-In" log on page 30 from Sarah's bootcamp regime as an example, you can keep track of your results on the blank log provided on page 31. Make photocopies so you can have multiple logs.

Real Brides: Tips from the Trenches

I took at least two friends with me every time I went to try wedding cakes or caterers. This way I could have only one bite of everything. It really takes only one bite to know if you like it or not. My friends added valuable input as I made my vendor choices. —*Recruit Susan*

Step One: Planning

No mission can be successful without a good plan of attack. Taking five minutes at the beginning of every week will guarantee that you will achieve your monthly and overall goals. Plan your exercise, plan your meals, and plan your success. Planning turns into progress, and that is what it is all about. Every week you are going to review your plan and your progress, make improvements, and move forward. That's a good soldier!

At the beginning of each week, take the time to plan out the next seven days. Make sure to plan your exercise and your nutrition before you go to the grocery store. And don't shop for food on an empty stomach.

Think about your weekly commitments, your schedule, and your exercise plan. In pen, put your exercise routine in your bootcamp plan. You are scheduling exercise just as you would schedule a meeting with potential caterers. For example, on Wednesday, recruit and bride-to-be Jessica does her strength training before work, because she usually has evening meetings with her wedding planner, and on Thursday nights she takes an hour-long kickboxing class at the gym because that's what her schedule allows.

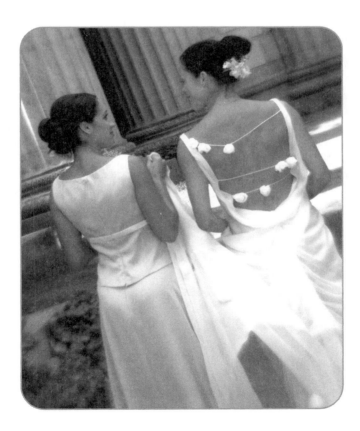

Report-In: Real Recruit Sarah

	MONTH SIX	MONTH FIVE	MONTH FOUR	MONTH THREE	MONTH TWO	MONTH ONE	WEDDING DAY
WEIGHT	**Goal:** Lose 5 pounds — 171 lbs	**Goal:** Lose 5 pounds — 166 lbs	**Goal:** Lose 5 pounds — 161 lbs	**Goal:** Lose 5 pounds — 156 lbs	**Goal:** Lose 5 pounds — 151 lbs	**Goal:** Lose 5 pounds — 146 lbs	**146 lbs**
	Report: 170 lbs Lost 6 pounds	**Report:** 165 lbs Lost 5 pounds	**Report:** 158 lbs Wow, lost 7 pounds	**Report:** 154 lbs Getting harder, lost 4 pounds	**Report:** 149 lbs Woo hoo, made it over the hump, lost 5 pounds	**Report:** 146 lbs *Did it!* Lost 3 pounds	
CLOTHING SIZE	**Goal:** 14 comfortably	**Goal:** 12	**Goal:** 10	**Goal:** 8	**Goal:** Maintain	**Goal:** Maintain	
	Report: 14	**Report:** 12	**Report:** 10, fit into some old jeans	**Report:** 8, can finally fit into every-thing in my closet	**Report:** Did it	**Report:** Not a problem	**Size 8**
FITNESS	**Goal:** Run 2 miles	**Goal:** Run 4 miles	**Goal:** Run 6 miles	**Goal:** Run 8 miles	**Goal:** Run 10K		
	Report: Tough but did it	**Report:** Felt great	**Report:** Wow! I rock	**Report:** Excellent. Will start swimming	**Report:** Got my T-shirt and medal. Signing up for triathlon		**Ran 12 miles**
INCHES	**Report:**	**Report:**	**Report:**	**Report:**	**Report:**	**Report:**	
ARM	12½	12¼	12	11¾	11½	11	**18 inches lost**
BUST	38	37	35	34	33	32	
WAIST	30	29½	28¾	28½	28	27	
HIPS	40	38	36¾	36¾	36	35½	
THIGH	25	24¼	23½	23½	23¼	22	

INCHES LOST: 1½ + 6 + 3 + 4½ + 3 = 18 INCHES

Report-In: Your Turn!

	MONTH SIX	MONTH FIVE	MONTH FOUR	MONTH THREE	MONTH TWO	MONTH ONE	WEDDING DAY
WEIGHT	Goal: Report:	Goal: Report:	Goal: Report:	Goal: Report:	Goal: Report:	Goal: Report:	
CLOTHING SIZE	Goal: Report:	Goal: Report:	Goal: Report:	Goal: Report:	Goal: Report:	Goal: Report:	
FITNESS	Goal: Report:	Goal: Report:	Goal: Report:	Goal: Report:	Goal: Report:	Goal: Report:	
INCHES ARM BUST WAIST HIPS THIGH	Report:	Report:	Report:	Report:	Report:	Report:	

➥ **INCHES LOST:**

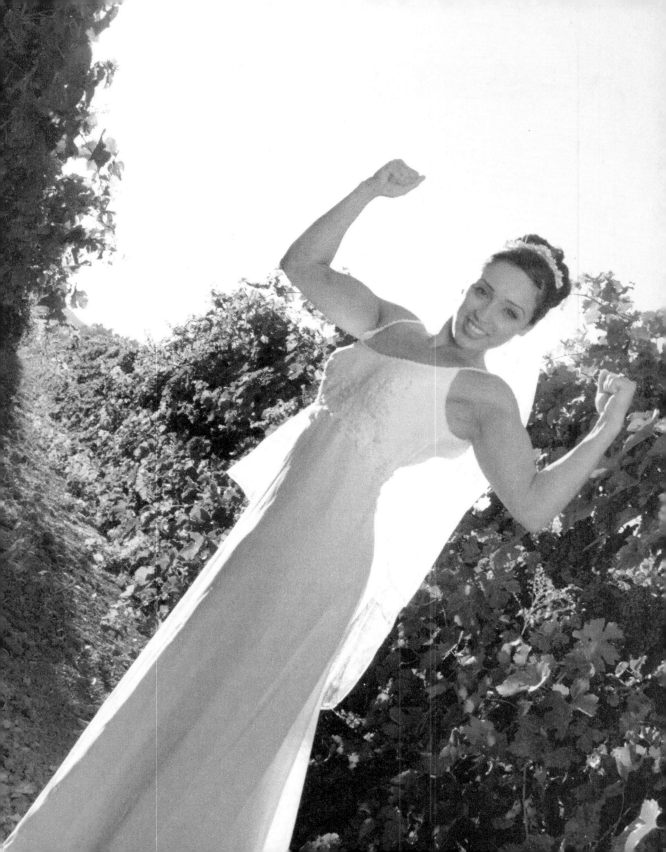

SOMETHING OLD

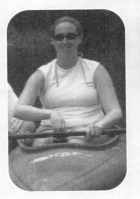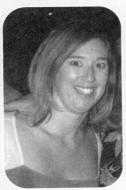

SOMETHING NEW

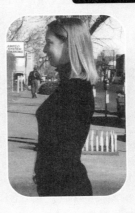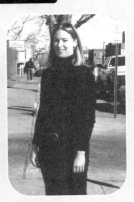

I felt fabulous, when I first tried on my wedding dress because I knew it was the perfect dress for me. But I felt huge, because the zipper on the size 4 sample dress wouldn't even begin to zip. And I felt silly when the woman from the store tried with all her might to pull the back of the dress closed so I could see how it would look if it fit correctly.

Before I started Bootcamp360, I looked and felt "big." I was fairly active, but I knew I wanted to be thinner, stronger, in better shape, and altogether healthier. Bootcamp360 helped me reach my goals by teaching me what I needed to alter in my lifestyle in order to be fit and healthy.

I felt so great when I started seeing results and even better when everyone around me noticed results. I needed that success to keep me motivated and I got it! First it was the jeans that were suddenly too big around the waist. Then it was all the energy I seemed to have all day long—no more afternoon lulls. The success just kept coming and coming. I still receive compliments every day. Friends who haven't seen me in a while rave about the way I look, and everyone wants to know what program I am on. There is really no better feeling than seeing friends again and having them almost not recognize you because you are so much trimmer and fitter than they have ever seen you.

I am now buying clothes that are three sizes smaller than when I started. I even fit into a pair of shorts from high school! It feels great to actually see yourself getting smaller and to see your trouble spots become less "troublesome." I have completely changed my eating habits and I work out regularly. Bootcamp has helped me maintain a regular regime, a healthy diet, and a positive self-image.

I know that a few months from now when I walk down the aisle, I will look the best I have ever looked (and felt).

Step Two: Progress

It's called moving into position. You've spent five minutes planning your exercise for the rest of the week. It's Sunday night and you now have all of these great plans. The real progress is made when you hold yourself accountable for putting those great plans into action. You will write down all the exercise you do get as well as everything you eat and drink. You must be honest with yourself here. Fibbing about it will only hurt your progress in the long run. Along with your food and exercise, you will write down any thoughts and comments for the day. Did you go an extra mile in your run? Was your group exercise class too easy today? Were you hungry all day? Did you have more energy today? All of your thoughts and comments are important for your progress as well.

Step Three: Review

Review your progress relative to your plan. Did you accomplish everything you said you would? If yes, congratulations and keep it up. If no, why not? Reviewing your progress will help you improve your efforts as you move forward. To plan for the future, you must first understand the past.

Having a bad week and can't figure out how to make it better? Simply pull out one of your "star logs" (a log from a really good day).

I DO #5: WEDDING PARTY BATTLE BUDDIES Along with keeping your "Report-In" exercise and "Plan and Progress" nutrition logs, battle buddies are a great way of holding you accountable. They will praise you for your accomplishments, whether it be choosing flattering bridesmaid dresses for all your friends or getting up early in the mornings to work out. Battle buddies will also call you out for eating cookies after dinner or using your busy work schedule as an excuse for not exercising. Most important, your battle buddies can provide inspiration when it's time to remotivate.

Enlist your bridesmaids, friends at work, your mom, or even your fiancé as your battle buddies. And on your special day, when you look and feel amazing, don't forget to give your battle buddies a special hug for helping you along.

CONGRATULATIONS! The checklist is complete, the equipment is ready. Now it's time to move out, soldier! **REMEMBER, THIS IS B-O-O-T-C-A-M-P.**

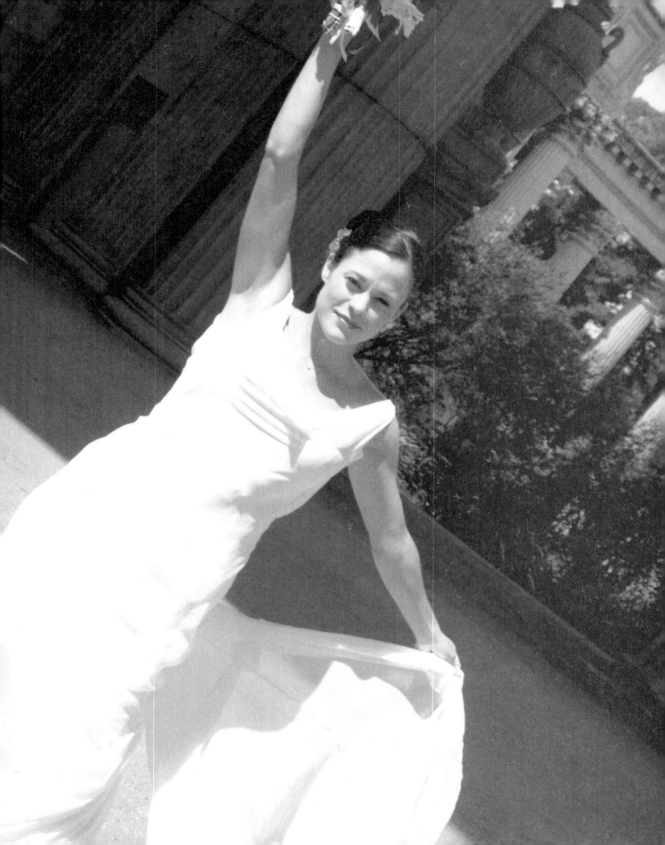

TRAINING BEGINS

How much time do you have to prepare for your big day and for your life to come? One year? Six months? Two months? Are you looking for steady results or are you in a time crunch? Bootcamp360 for Brides is designed to fit in wherever you are in your engagement cycle. It is optimal to begin at least six months before your wedding, but we recognize that every bride and situation is different.

Follow these guidelines to get the most out of the bootcamp regime. Regardless of your starting point, the program will ensure that you are his better half, not his better three-quarters. March on, soldier!

EQUIPMENT

Exercise equals movement, and movement equals a tight, toned bride. Bootcamp360 is going to arm you with all the gear you need to succeed. No excuses! Before you start sculpting your body, read through this section and spend some time preparing your barracks.

Exercise will ensure that your arms, legs, and back are lean and toned as you frolic in the water with your new husband (get used to saying it). You need to get out of that chair and off that couch and expend more calories. Your mission, and you will accept it, is to make exercise your second love—next to your husband of course.

The equipment below is everything you need to perform all the exercises—aerobic, strength, and flexibility.

- **Resistance band**
- **Jump rope**
- **Exercise ball**
- **3 sets of free weights (low, medium, high)**
  - **If you are new to free weights: 4 lbs, 8 lbs, and 12 lbs**
  - **If you have lifted before: 8 lbs, 12 lbs, and 15 lbs**
- **A good workout outfit**
- **Exercise logs (see page 232)**

RESISTANCE BAND

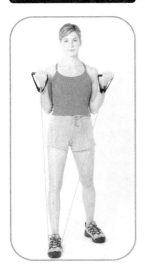

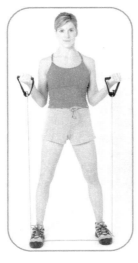

The resistance band is an integral part of this program: You will use it for everything from strength training to abdominal work to flexibility. Buy one that is durable and has handles.

One great benefit of a resistance band is that you can vary the difficulty of an exercise simply by decreasing the amount of tubing you have to use. For example, you can increase the difficulty of a bicep curl or similar exercises by standing on the band with both feet instead of just one, giving you less band to pull on. You can increase the level of difficulty in a chest press or similar exercises by placing your hands closer together on the band. This applies to all exercises with the resistance band. Just as with your free weights, the last three to four of thirty repetitions with the resistance band should be difficult to complete. Play around with it your first few workouts to find the right level of difficulty for you. You can always adjust the difficulty as you exercise.

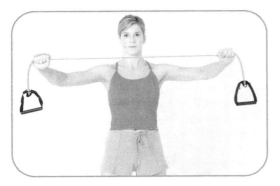

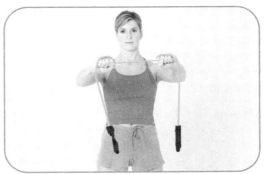

JUMP ROPE

Jumping rope is one of the best calorie-burning activities you can do, giving you the best overall workout in the shortest amount of time. If you are not yet ready for a high-intensity aerobic workout, don't worry. You will get there. Your progress will really impress and help motivate you even more. It's also perfect for days when you run out of time for your longer workouts or have extra time to spare. I always tell my recruits to jump rope for fifteen minutes on the days they simply can't work out. Jump ropes (and resistance bands) are also the perfect travel companion, taking almost no space in your suitcase. Now you have no excuse for not exercising when you are traveling or really busy.

When choosing a jump rope, you are better off buying one that is too long versus too short. As in the photo, the handles of the jump rope should come up to your armpits. If you need to shorten the rope, simply tie a single knot on each side below the handles.

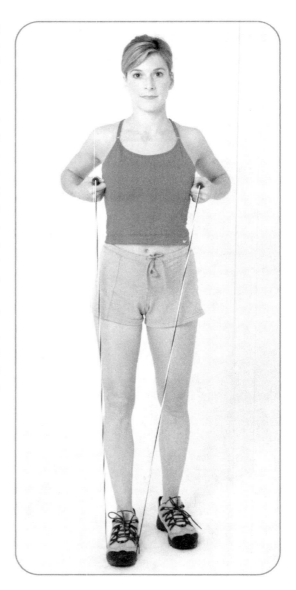

EXERCISE BALL

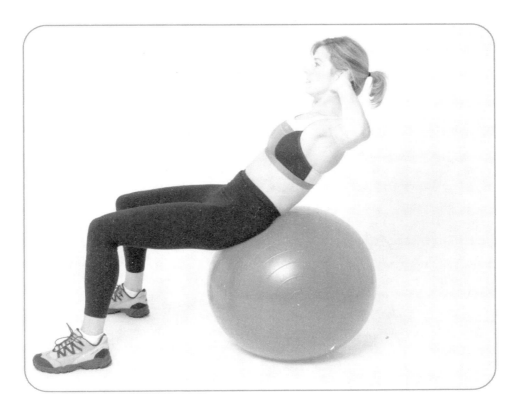

The exercise ball is at the core of the Bootcamp360 strength-training and flexibility workouts. The exercise ball uses multiple muscles just as any other activity: walking, speaking, going up stairs, etc. A lot of gym equipment isolates one muscle or muscle group at a time, but this is not how our bodies operate in real life. Bootcamp360 believes your workouts should reflect how your body really works, engaging (no pun intended) several muscles at one time.

Doing workouts on the exercise ball forces you to use multiple muscle groups to balance and stabilize the body while performing a specific task. For example, doing abdominal crunches on the ball engages not only the abdominal muscles performing the task, but your legs for balance and your core muscles for stability. With the exercise ball, you get a more thorough workout every time. As you step up in the bootcamp levels, you will incorporate the exercise ball more and more.

FREE WEIGHTS

You will need three sets of free weights for the duration of this program. I recommend buying light, medium, and heavy sets. Your weights will most likely include a set of four, eight, and twelve pounds or a set of eight, twelve, and fifteen pounds. You can always replace your weights with lower or higher weights depending on your strength and progress.

Different muscle groups will be able to lift varying amounts and therefore require different levels of weights. For example, the latissimus dorsi in your back, due to its size and configuration, can lift more weight than your triceps (back of your upper arms). And your leg muscles can accommodate a lot more weight than your shoulder muscles.

As you get stronger, you will want to increase your weights. If you find that the twelve-pound weights are getting too easy, you only need to buy a set of fifteen-pound weights to kick it up a notch.

When buying weights, try a few exercises from the program either at the gym or at the store before you make a purchase. This will help you determine the right weights for you. As with the resistance band, the weights you pick should make the last seven or eight of thirty repetitions difficult to complete. Hup to it—you should feel the burn!

A GOOD WORKOUT OUTFIT   This is partially indulgent but definitely worth it. You may be comfortable in a baggy T-shirt and track pants, but you probably won't feel like an athlete-in-training if you look like you're ready to crash on the couch. A good workout outfit that makes you feel fit and confident can make all the difference. It's really motivating to see the muscles that you're working and know that your movements are making a difference. Go ahead, go shopping. Also make sure to get a good pair of shoes, especially for your aerobic workouts. The right ones can help prevent injury to your joints and body.

Real Brides: **Tips from the Trenches**

Spend time with your fiancé that is more meaningful than mindlessly vegging on the couch and watching television. Go for a walk around the block, run in the park, or even work out at the gym together. It's a great way to get some extra exercise in before your day ends, and you will be amazed at what you learn about each other.

EXERCISE OVERVIEW

You are a soldier in love and with a mission. So give your fiancé a passionate kiss, change into your exercise clothes, and start sweating. In fact, exercise and love have a lot in common. Both make your heart rate jump, they increase your feelings of self-confidence, and they release feel-good hormones.

As a bride-to-be your days are packed full of meetings with vendors, family phone calls, and perusing magazines for ideas—not to mention your job and spending quiet time with your fiancé. In only thirty to sixty minutes a day, six days a week, Bootcamp360 will fit right into your schedule.

Just as all the elements of your wedding work together as one to create the perfect event, so do all the exercises work to create a toned, fit body. This program combines the right balance of aerobic, strength, and flexibility training to ensure the maximum amount of results. In Bootcamp360 we believe in the following balance: 50 percent cardio, 40 percent strength training, and 10 percent flexibility. Each of these elements is an equally important piece in your overall fitness.

The right balance of these three elements will quickly, safely, and effectively propel you toward your goals and your dress. Strength training increases muscle mass, which in turn increases your daily metabolism. This is crucial because muscle is the furnace that burns fat continually. Also, strength or resistance training puts stresses on your bones, which in turn strengthens them. This decreases the chances of osteoporosis (brittle bones) as we age, which is especially important for us better halves.

Aerobic exercise burns the fat stored just under your skin and improves your cardiovascular health. Flexibility keeps joints healthy, prevents injury, and helps develop long and lean muscles.

You need each of these—strength, aerobic activity, and flexibility—to build a solid and toned gown-worthy body. As fitness improves, your energy will soar, and what once seemed out of reach, such as spending the day hiking, will be close at hand. You will find that feelings of tiredness and lethargy decrease dramatically as your body becomes accustomed to doing more with less effort. Without a doubt, this increase in fitness contributes to energy expenditure and weight loss and control.

The important thing to remember is that the sooner you start, the sooner you accomplish your goals. This is important especially as you approach the wedding. Just think, if you accomplish your goals two months prior to your wedding date, your mental energy can be focused on maintaining your weight and fitness (which is much easier than losing) and, more important, finishing up the details of the most important day of your life.

Your Bootcamp360 exercise regime includes four days of aerobic exercise, two days of strength and flexibility work, and one "day pass." Each workout should consist of thirty to sixty minutes of continual exercise.

Let's go over each element separately and in more detail. It is important that you understand not only what you need to do, but also why you need to do it.

Real Brides: Tips from the Trenches

The veil is meant to hide your face, not your rear side. To ensure a toned rear side, do lunges in the kitchen and wall squats while you brush your teeth. —*Recruit Katie*

STRENGTH TRAINING

Unlike fat, muscle is active and continues to burn fat even when you aren't exercising. Anaerobic activity, meaning without oxygen, uses glycogen as its main fuel source. Lactic acid, the by-product of glycogen use, causes the soreness you feel the day after your workout. Anaerobic activity helps you build muscle, therefore increasing your basal metabolic rate. This is the rate at which energy is used by an organism at rest, typically measured in calories released per kilogram of body weight. A direct correlation exists between muscle mass and basal metabolic rate. Simply put, the more muscle you have, the more calories you burn on any given day. Proper strength training has also been proven to increase aerobic stamina and ability. This is mostly due to the increase in lean muscle that is available for aerobic work.

Strength training is going to give you that toned, lean look you want on your wedding day, es-

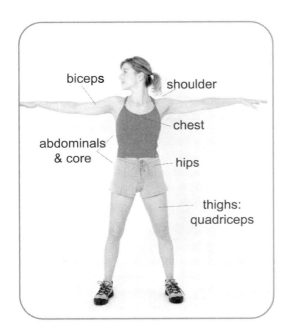

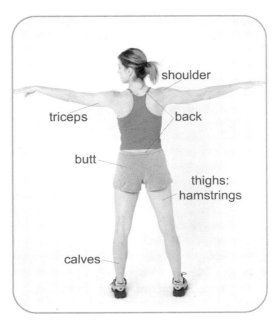

pecially in your arms and upper body. Bootcamp360 strength training is designed specially with this in mind. This type of strength training has an endurance base, ensuring that you build strength without building bulk. Endurance is achieved by repetitive contractions of the muscles, which requires continuous energy supplies, and your strength is built by lifting heavy weights over a short period. As women and as brides our goal is to look toned, not bulky. This is achieved through lower weights and more repetitions (that is, the number of times you repeat an exercise).

As outlined in the workouts, you will perform thirty repetitions for each exercise and then, without rest, move on to the next exercise. The routines begin with the lower body and work their way up the body, completing all muscle groups. This creates a strength-training routine that will build strength without bulk. Don't get me wrong—muscle will appear and your biceps will be defined, but you will look sexy and feminine, not huge and hulky.

First-time recruits often struggle with their strength-training routine during the first week or so. This is natural and to be expected. In fact, I expect you not to be able to complete all thirty repetitions on your first few attempts. Each time, push yourself to add a few more repetitions until you eventually reach thirty. Continue at that level and with the weight if the last six to eight of thirty repetitions are still pushing you to work hard. Like any good soldier in basic training, you'll feel the burn and learn to love it!

If you have thumbed through the workout photos, you have noticed that there are multiple abdominal exercises. Your abdominals are a combination of smaller muscles that vary in size and direction. To see results in the troublesome midsection of your body, you need to perform a range of abdominal exercises. For example, regular crunches work the front and upper portions of your abdominals, while side toe touches work the sides and lower portions of your abdominals. Furthermore, you must be diligent about your aerobic workouts if you want to see the "six-pack" hiding underneath. Aerobic workouts are what burn the fat, particularly in the middle, and the strength exercises are what define the muscles. This is true for your entire body, but it is particularly true for your midsection.

AEROBIC ACTIVITY

Aerobic activity is what will help you burn the fat that covers the muscles you are building through strength training. Have you ever heard someone complain that they still don't look toned even after lifting weights? The reason is that without aerobic fat-burning exercise, those muscles will remain buried in fat. Also, aerobic activity increases your overall fitness level and health. Below is a description of exactly what aerobic activity is so that you achieve the maximum effects.

Say that you start your step class at a slow rate to warm up. You are not yet sweating or breathing hard. After about five minutes you pick up the intensity, sweating and breathing hard but keeping up. At this point, you are in the "fat-burning zone," which means "in the presence of oxygen." The energy you are using is the oxidation of fat and carbohydrates in your body. This is aerobic activity. Aerobic activity, meaning "with oxygen," is extremely important for cardiovascular and pulmonary health. Walking, running, biking, and kickboxing are just some examples of aerobic exercise.

Then, the instructor tells you to push it, and you feel your breathing become labored and shallow and it feels as if you can't continue. Now you are at a point where you can no longer continue and have transitioned your workout into the anaerobic zone, previously discussed. This is evident by the presence of lactic acid, which means that you are burning energy faster than you can produce it aerobically. While that is appropriate for strength, it is not the goal of aerobic activity.

Aerobic exercise's main source of fuel is fat, mostly the subcutaneous fat, nestled underneath your skin. Correct intensity of aerobic activity puts you in the fat-burning zone while you exercise. In the fat-burning zone you are continually providing the body with the oxygen it needs to burn fat and carbohydrates. Aerobic exercise is what will get rid of the excess fat on your abdominals and the rest of your body.

Fat is the most abundant source of energy. Each pound of fat is equal to 3,500 calories. If a recruit weighs 170 pounds and has 28 percent body fat, she is carrying around 47.6 pounds of fat. That means that this recruit has 166,600 calories of energy stored in her body. Considering that the average woman burns 100 calories per mile while jogging, she has enough energy stored up to run 1,666 miles. Therefore, almost all of us have the stores we need to burn fat during exercise, so it benefits you greatly to train your body into becoming a fat-burning machine.

At first your body is presented with a challenge, but as your fitness level increases, activities that once seemed tough will become easier. As with your measurements and your weight, this challenge becomes the benchmark by which your progress will be measured. Your mission may range from exercising for the first time, adding fifteen minutes to your aerobic routine, or trying a new routine. When presented with this task, your body has to work harder than usual to step up and accomplish it. Your body does this by pumping more blood to your muscles, sweating harder, and tapping into fat stores for energy. Your body will continue to work hard as long as your aerobic workouts are challenging.

We want our bodies to be fat-burning machines. Using the "talk test" and the "aerobic heart rate" charts will help you measure the intensity of the exercise and make sure that you are staying within the "zone" and continuing to see results. Your aerobic workouts should always be within the 6 to 8 range on both the talk-test and the heart-rate charts. Lower than 6 is too easy and higher than 8 puts you in the anaerobic zone, where you are no longer using fat as your main fuel source.

The talk test, below, measures your rate of exertion, or how hard you are working out. Many times our perceived rate of how hard we think we are working out is not accurate. Don't just guess, take the test. Knowing that you need to be between 6 and 8, try to hold a conversation (even with yourself) every so often during your workout. If you can hold a full conversation, you are not working out hard enough. If you can talk but must take pauses to breathe or are only able to speak with short sentences, you are in the zone. If you have reached a point where you simply can't talk and your breathing is quick and shallow, you need to decrease the intensity and get yourself back to burning fat.

10 — Can't talk
9
8 — Can answer someone briefly but not hold a full conversation
7
6 — Can talk with pauses to breathe every few sentences
5
4 — Able to hold a full conversation while exercising
3
2
1 — Sitting on the couch engaged in a full conversation

Another great way to make sure you are within the aerobic or fat-burning zone is to check your heart rate. For an efficient aerobic workout you should be at approximately 60 to 80 percent (6 to 8) of your maximum heart rate. As with the talk test, this is the optimal aerobic range for fat-burning. At 6 to 8 you are pumping more blood through your body and delivering greater amounts of oxygen to working muscles. A good estimate of your maximum heart rate is 220 minus your age. Review the chart and do the calculations to find your fat-burning zone.

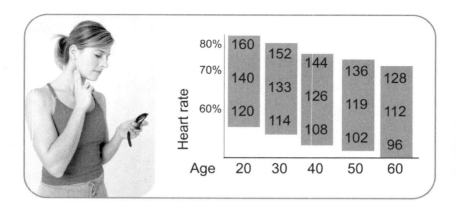

If you are new to fitness, focus on getting your heart rate in the 6 and 7 range. As you improve, you can increase that focus to the 7 and 8 range. If you are a seasoned athlete, focus on continually achieving a 7 to 8 range.

It is crucial that you check your heart rate periodically as you exercise. I encourage you to buy a heart-rate monitor to make this even easier. If you don't, you can easily take your own heart rate. To take your heart rate, put your index and your middle finger against your neck in the indent just below your jawline. You should be able to easily find your pulse here. Count your heart rate for twenty seconds and multiply by three. This will give you your heart rate per minute and allow you to check your level using the chart above.

After you warm up for five minutes at an easy pace, such as by walking on the treadmill or jumping rope lightly, your goal is to maintain the fat-burning zone for the remainder of your work-out until you are ready to cool down and stretch.

In aerobic exercise, intensity and duration are inversely related. This means that to burn the same number of calories you have to work out twice as long walking as you do running. Don't let this scare you into focusing only on high-intensity exercises. Many types and styles of aerobic work-outs have been created, and each has its merits and benefits. Aerobic exercises such as running, step class, jumping rope, and skiing are high intensity. While these exercises burn the most calories per hour, they are also harder on the joints. They require a high level of impact, especially on the knee joint. Exercises such as the elliptical machine, brisk walking, and biking are slightly lower in intensity and are much kinder on the joints. However, they do not burn as many calories per hour. The lower-intensity exercises such as swimming and low-impact aerobics classes are especially suited for those who either cannot place that type of stress on the joints or are simply not accustomed to exercise yet. Lastly, find exercises that you find challenging *and* fun.

220 – age = _____ (maximum heart rate)

- Maximum heart rate x .80 = _____ (8—top range of fat-burning zone)
- Maximum heart rate x .70 = _____ (7—midrange of fat-burning zone)
- Maximum heart rate x .60 = _____ (6—low range of fat-burning zone)

ACTIVITY	CALORIES/MINUTE
Sleeping	1.2
Sitting, reading	1.3
Standing	1.5
Walking indoors	3.1
House painting	3.5
Sweeping floors	3.9
Gardening, weeding	5.6
Shoveling snow	7.1
Walking up stairs	15
Rowing, vigorous	15
Cycling, easy	5
Cycling, vigorous	15
Mountain climbing	15
Martial arts	13
Skiing, moderate	8
Skiing, steep	20
Swimming, leisurely	6
Swimming, vigorous	12.5
Dancing	6
Walking, flat	6
Walking uphill, 15% grade	20
Hiking with backpack	6.8
Jogging, 12-min mile	10
Running, 6-min mile	20

The chart above gives you the average amount of calories used per minute for various exercises, including both daily activities around the house and vigorous exercises. Notice how the calorie expenditure increases with intensity. Think about this as well as you pick your aerobic activities.

If you are new to exercise, it is recommended that you begin with the lower-intensity exercises and eventually work your way up to the higher-intensity ones. If you are used to running, try a different high-intensity exercise such as indoor group cycling or kickboxing.

Here is an example of what your aerobic progression may look like over four weeks' time:

Week 1	Week 2	Week 3	Week 4
• Kickboxing, 45 minutes —range 8 • Walk for 30 minutes —range 7 • Bootcamp360 Basic	• Kickboxing, 45 minutes—range 7 • Walk for 45 minutes —range 7 • Bootcamp360 Basic	• Kickboxing, 60 minutes—range 8 • Walk for 45 minutes, jog for last 5 minutes— range 8 • Bootcamp360 Basic	• Kickboxing, 60 minutes, and 5 minutes jumping rope —range 7 • Walk for 45 minutes, jog for last 10 minutes —range 8 • Bootcamp360 Advanced

As you can see from the chart above, this recruit maintained her goal of keeping within the 6 to 8 range by increasing her time and eventually her intensity.

As you continue on with the same task, your body becomes more and more efficient and no longer needs to work as hard to accomplish the same results. As you progress, you will notice that your heart rate will actually decrease while performing the same exercise. More than likely you won't sweat as much and it becomes much easier to breathe. This is not only normal, but also a good sign that you are becoming more fit. However, if you continue exercising while un-challenged, you will plateau. A plateau basically means that you are exercising without progress-ing forward. This is where you stop seeing results. To any good bootcamp recruit a plateau is unacceptable!

To keep improving, your aerobic activity must increase in intensity to stay in the fat-burning zone. To do this, add some quick sprints to your runs, ride faster on your bike, and walk at a greater incline. Another way of stepping it up is to change your routine—add a day of swimming, switch from step class to cardio boxing, bike instead of walk. You can also add time to your routine—go the extra mile, swim the extra lap, stay after your cardio class and get on the tread-mill for ten minutes. You don't want your body to stop improving once it becomes accustomed to your workouts.

Either pick one of the exercises listed below or add your own. New exercises come out all the time, so feel free to experiment. If you are fairly new to aerobic exercise or have taken a lot of time off from your workouts, pick a low-intensity activity such as swimming or walking. If you are fairly active but somewhat inconsistent in your workouts, pick medium-intensity workouts such as the el-liptical machine or biking. If you are aerobically fit and already regularly do medium- and high-intensity workouts, pick new high-intensity workouts such as indoor group cycling and hill hiking.

I also recommend picking new activities as you move up the bootcamp levels. You'll be challenging yourself continually, and you may even discover a new workout that you enjoy. Bootcamp360 is for women who want results, so pick your aerobic exercises with the mind-set of an army private, not a lethargic couch potato. Avoid the path of least resistance at all costs!

Low Intensity	Medium Intensity	High Intensity
Swimming	Elliptical machine	Running
Water aerobics	StairMaster	Indoor group cycling
Water walking	Dance lessons	Boxing
Walking	Flat hiking	Cardio kickboxing
Low-impact aerobics	Biking (indoor & outdoor)	Cardio chisel
Neurokinetics	In-line skating	Martial arts
Beginner yoga	Snowshoeing	Jump rope
Yard work/gardening	Cross-country skiing	Kayaking
Horseback riding	Rowing machine	Skiing
Other _____	Yoga*	Snowboarding
	Tennis	Step aerobics
	Other _____	Hill hiking
		Yoga*
		Other _____

* Depends on style and instructor

It is extremely important that you warm up prior to elevating your aerobic intensity. Warming up will prepare your body for what's to come by deepening your breathing, pumping more blood through the body, and delivering more oxygen to the muscles. Your warm-up should consist of five minutes at a low intensity. Doing a moderate walk on the treadmill, performing jumping jacks, and lightly jumping rope are great warm-ups. Before you kick it up a notch, gently stretch the major lower-body muscle groups (quadriceps, hamstrings, and calves). Preventing injury is key here.

Also, take your heart rate halfway through your exercise when your body is efficiently warmed up to determine the degree of difficulty. If you picked in-line skating to start and find it too difficult, change your plan to include swimming or low-impact aerobics or slow down your pace. If you found the elliptical machine too easy, move up to a high-intensity exercise like cardio kickboxing or jumping rope.

Real Brides: Tips from the Trenches

I walk for exercise. To keep motivated, I started visualizing myself walking down the aisle. I walk around the block as if it is my wedding day: shoulders back, head up, and perfect posture. —*Recruit Danielle*

FLEXIBILITY

The third element in fitness is stretching and flexibility. Stretching prepares the body's nervous system, increases the temperature of muscles, and helps prevent injury to joints and muscles. Flexibility promotes good posture and circulation. Flexibility also allows for full range of motion in your joints, causing your body to perform aerobic and strength-training activities with a wide range of motion.

Stretching is an integral part of warming up and cooling down. You should do a few minutes of stretching after you have warmed up on the treadmill or bike for at least five minutes. Think of your muscles as Silly Putty. When you first take Silly Putty out of the eggshell and pull it apart, it breaks. The Silly Putty is cold, just like your muscles when you start to work out. When you start to play with the Silly Putty, it warms up and you can stretch it across the room without breaking it. This is how your muscles work.

Your major flexibility work will occur at the end of your strength workout, when your muscles are warm. This is when your muscles and your joints will benefit the most. This also gives your heart rate a chance to recover slowly. You will hold each stretching pose statically for at least thirty seconds so that you get the maximum benefit. No bouncing! Static stretching involves slow, fluid movements to reach the point of stretch. Gently work your way into the pose, going deeper into the stretch on your exhales. This doesn't need to be painful, but you do need to feel the stretch.

Begin your strength and flexibility training routines with Bootcamp360 Basic. You will be doing Basic two times a week, with at least one day of aerobics or rest in between.

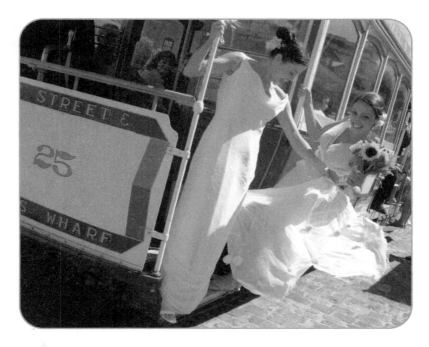

More than likely as you move up in bootcamp levels, you will have to decrease your weights to accommodate harder exercises. This is because the specific exercises in each level are harder and require more work from your muscles. You didn't think we would keep the exercise easy as you got closer to your wedding, did you?

For example, in Basic you will do backward lunges with weights. In Advanced, you will do backward lunges with weights, adding a knee lift. In Hard Core, you will do backward lunges with weights and a knee up, adding alternating punches. This applies to all the exercises you will perform. Adding a knee up makes the exercise harder to execute. It takes more muscle coordination and engages more of your core muscles for balance.

Here's a brief overview of Basic, Advanced, and Hard Core, giving you a basic understanding of what each level entails. The charts below offer examples of a one-year, six-month, and three-month recruit in training.

Real Brides: Tips from the Trenches

Avoid distracting tan lines on your wedding day. Instead of sun worshipping, which actually ages the skin, try a self-tanning lotion. But be sure to apply it a few days before your wedding. You don't want it to run all over your crisp white wedding dress.

Engagement Exercise Schedule

1 YEAR

Month 12	Month 11	Month 10	Month 9	Month 8	Month 7	Month 6	Month 5	Month 4	Month 3	Month 2	Month 1
BASIC				ADVANCED				HARD CORE			
WEDDING WEEK											
BRIDE'S 1-HOUR WORKOUT (SEE PAGE 157)											

6 MONTHS

Month 6	Month 5	Month 4	Month 3	Month 2	Month 1
BASIC		ADVANCED		HARD CORE	
WEDDING WEEK					
BRIDE'S 1-HOUR WORKOUT (SEE PAGE 157)					

3 MONTHS

Month 3	Month 2	Month 1	Wedding Week
BASIC	ADVANCED	HARD CORE	BRIDE'S 1-HOUR WORK-OUT (SEE PAGE 157)

BASIC STRENGTH AND FLEXIBILITY

Basic is all about getting your body moving and making exercise a part of your daily routine. Your strength and flexibility workout is a full-body routine working all angles of your body, to be performed two days a week, in between your aerobic workouts. You will work all your major muscle groups: legs (thighs, hips, and butt), calves, back, chest, shoulders, biceps, triceps, and abdominals. When you have completed your strength training, you will hold each flexibility pose for at least thirty seconds.

ADVANCED STRENGTH AND FLEXIBILITY

Advanced is all about challenging your body and increasing your efforts. The strength and flexibility training routine is a challenging full-body routine that features more abdominals and core work. Great core and abdominal muscles are the key to good posture as you glide down the aisle and pose for the wedding photographer. Your routines will now use the exercise ball even more. On

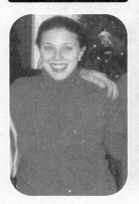
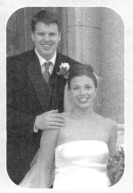
every exhale make it a point to go deeper into your flexibility poses than before, continuing to hold each pose for at least thirty seconds.

HARD CORE STRENGTH AND FLEXIBILITY

At this point, you are getting close to your wedding, and we want to make sure that every workout counts. Now we will add even more upper-body exercises to your strength-training routine, especially for the triceps and back. We want to make sure that you have lean, toned arms and upper

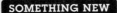
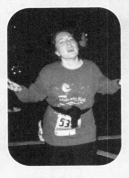
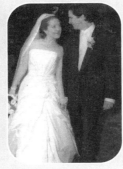
body as you take your husband's arms for your first dance as a married couple. In other words, we want to see you sweat! The flexibility poses will accentuate the trim, fit body you have sculpted over the past several months.

In "Bootcamp360 Resources" at the end of this book you will also find logs for each of the workouts above. I can't emphasize enough the importance of charting your workouts. I knew a woman who lifted weights at least four times a week, but she never saw much progress. I asked her the specifics

Real Brides: Tips from the Trenches

Get ready for your first dance as husband and wife and shed weight at the same time. Take waltz, swing, or even salsa lessons for your big debut as Mr. and Mrs., and wow your guests with your suave dance skills.

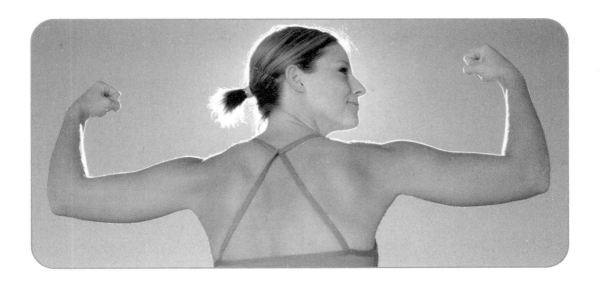

of her weight training. She told me that it really depended on the day and her mood. Some days she used ten pounds for the squats, other days fifteen pounds. Sometimes it was four pounds for the shoulder press, others it was eight pounds.

Do you see the problem? By lack of consistency she wasn't challenging her body at all. Some days were hard, some days were easy, and some days she simply went through the motions. You need to know if eight pounds is the right weight for your lateral raises or if it is too easy, demanding that you increase the weight to ten pounds. You also need to know how long you have been at the same level. If you have been lifting the same weight for the same exercise for over a month, it could tell you something important about your workouts. It could mean that you aren't consistent, or it could mean that you aren't pushing yourself and are simply going through the motions, which will not help you achieve your goals. If you cheat your workout, you're only cheating yourself.

You are cordially invited, at this very moment, to get your butt into shape . . . *now, soldier!*

Real Brides: Tips from the Trenches

Work travel usually means long days in conferences. With only four months to go before my wedding I simply wasn't willing to give up a week of my routine. This time I took advantage of my surroundings. I used my morning workouts as an opportunity to sightsee and enjoy the fresh outdoors. So the next time you travel, instead of getting frustrated, go for a speed walk and do some push-ups and triceps dips on the park bench. —*Recruit Sally*

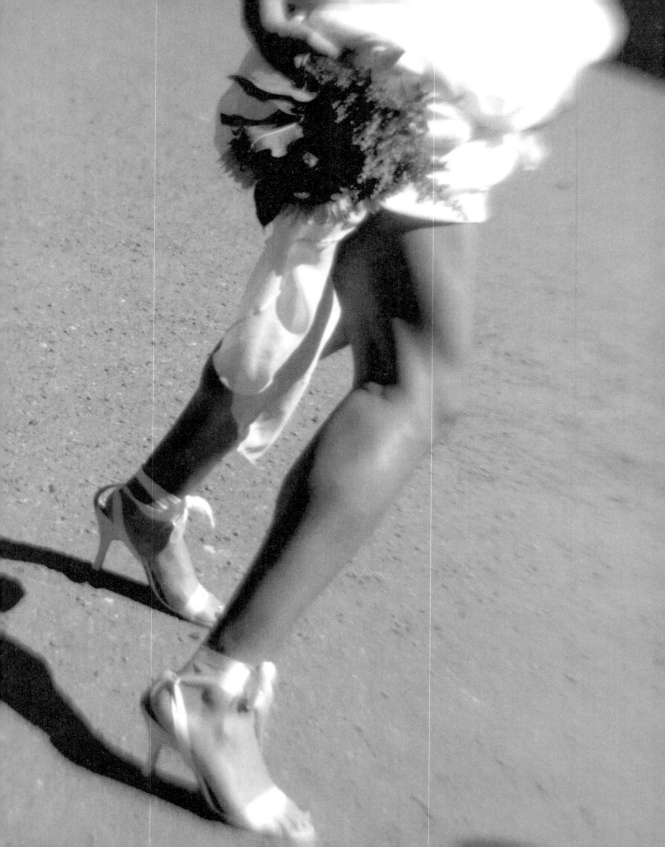

BOOTCAMP360
REGIMES

BASIC

At this point in your wedding planning you are most likely ripping out photos for inspiration and creative direction. You have probably spent endless hours showing off your sparkling ring and retelling everyone you know the romantic tale of your proposal. It's now time to stop talking and start taking action.

From the aerobic activity list on page 53, pick two exercises to commit to thirty to sixty minutes a day, four days a week. At this stage you should pick exercises that reflect your current fitness level. You don't want to burn out before you gain momentum, so if you are not accustomed to exercising, pick exercises that are low impact, such as swimming, walking, or low-impact aerobics. If you already do a lot of aerobic exercise, pick medium- or high-intensity workouts.

Your strength-training routine will get you accustomed to lifting free weights and building lean, healthy muscle. Along with the full-body strength training, your routine also includes yoga-inspired flexibility exercises. It is important that you do not skimp on this part of the routine. The flexibility exercises cool down the body, while increasing joint flexibility and preventing injury. Be diligent about holding each stretch for at least thirty seconds before moving on to the next pose. Dedicate two days each week to your full-body strength and flexibility routine. Spread these days out between your aerobic activities.

This book includes instructional photos and written descriptions of all the exercises you will perform. Use these photos to ensure that your form is correct and that you are getting the most out of each exercise. Use the correlating strength-training logs in "Bootcamp360 Resources" at the end of this book to track your progress.

Once Basic no longer presents a challenge (you have increased the weights several times and the aerobic exercise is easy) or you begin to plateau, step up to Advanced. This is usually after one and a half to two months of Basic.

Here is an example of what your week might look like:

MONDAY	TUESDAY	WEDNESDAY	THURSDAY	FRIDAY	SATURDAY	SUNDAY
Aerobic Kickboxing 45 minutes	*Strength & Flexibility* Basic workout	*Aerobic* Walking 60 minutes	*Strength & Flexibility* Basic workout	*Aerobic* Kickboxing 45–60 minutes	*Aerobic* Walking 60 minutes	Day Pass

Here are a few reasons why your week will follow the above example:

1. You need to accumulate enough aerobic exercise to train your body to become a fat-burning machine. This isn't going to be accomplished by doing aerobics only once or twice a week. Four days a week adds up to, at the minimum, two hours of aerobic, fat-burning exercises a week.

2. Switching your aerobic activities will keep them fun and challenging. Doing the same thing every day can be extremely boring. This way we are also decreasing the chances of plateauing quickly. Aerobic activity can be hard on the joints, and breaking up your week with strength training will help prevent injury.

3. Strength and flexibility routines will work all major muscle groups: legs (thighs, hips, and butt), calves, back, chest, shoulders, biceps, triceps, and abdominals. After a day of strength and flexibility, you want to give your body a rest from strength training and let it repair itself. When strength training, you tear your muscle fibers. It is the repair of these fibers in those twenty-four hours when you gain strength. Allowing your body to repair is an integral part of getting stronger and is as necessary as the exercise itself.

Notice that you always get one "day pass" a week. Honor that day. It is as important as the other six days. Giving yourself a day off, mentally and physically, helps prevent burnout and giving in to unnecessary cravings.

STRENGTH AND FLEXIBILITY

EXERCISE	MUSCLE GROUP
Warm-up	5 minutes: treadmill, bike, or jumping rope
Stretch	2 minutes: all major muscle groups
Backward Lunge	Legs
Plié Squat	Legs
Hamstring Roll with Arms Out	Legs
Inner-Thigh Exercise Ball Squeeze	Legs
Outer-Thigh Half-Moon	Legs
Standing Calf Raise	Calves
Knee Swimmer	Back
Standing Front Raise	Back
One-Arm Exercise Ball Row	Back
Knee Push-up	Chest
Chest Press on Exercise Ball	Chest
Resistance-Band Pull	Chest
Standing Overhead Press with Band	Shoulders
Standing Lateral Raise	Shoulders
Standing Biceps Curl	Biceps
Hammer Curl with Band	Biceps
Knee Triceps Push-up	Triceps
Standing Triceps Press	Triceps
Exercise Ball Crunch One	Abdominals
Bike on Floor	Abdominals
Dead Bug	Abdominals
Floor Oblique	Abdominals
Exercise Ball Push-Out	Abdominals
Side Toe Touch	Abdominals
Plank	Core
Downward Dog	Flexibility
Spinal Twist	Flexibility
Pigeon	Flexibility
Quadriceps Stretch	Flexibility
Hamstring Stretch	Flexibility
Calf Stretch	Flexibility
Chest and Biceps Stretch	Flexibility
Shoulder Stretch	Flexibility
Triceps Stretch	Flexibility

Perform each exercise, beginning with the backward lunges and completing your strength training with flexibility poses. Your goal is to perform thirty repetitions of each exercise. Don't worry if you can only do fifteen, twenty, or twenty-five. It is supposed to be challenging, and you will get to thirty as you get stronger. Once you complete an exercise, move on to the next without stopping. No time to waste!

BACKWARD LUNGE

Stand straight with both feet facing forward, arms holding weights at your sides. Keeping your upper body straight, place your leg straight behind you, far enough back to perform a lunge. Dip straight down, bending both knees. Do not let your front knee go beyond your ankle. Lift straight up, bringing your back leg back to starting position. Repeat on other side.

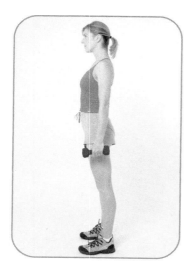 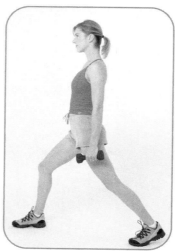 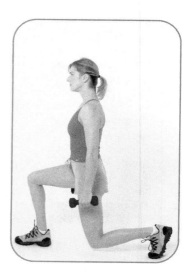

PLIÉ SQUAT

Place legs apart, wider than hip width, feet slightly turned out. Balance the weights on your shoulders with your hands, palms facing down. Bend into the squat, sticking your butt out as if you are trying to sit on a chair that is too far behind you. Bring your chest to your thighs as you bend down. Do not let your knees go beyond your ankles. Squeezing your butt muscles, lift yourself back to starting position.

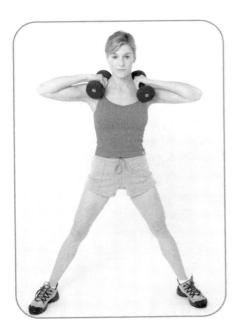
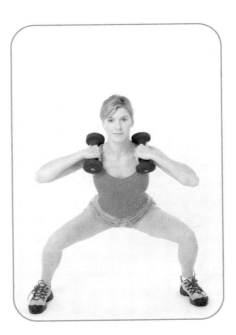

HAMSTRING ROLL WITH ARMS OUT

Lie flat on the floor with the heels of your feet on the ball and your arms flat out beside you. To begin, lift your torso off the floor creating a straight plank with your body. Using your hamstring and calf muscles, pull the ball toward you, keeping your upper body straight. With control, bring the ball back to its original position.

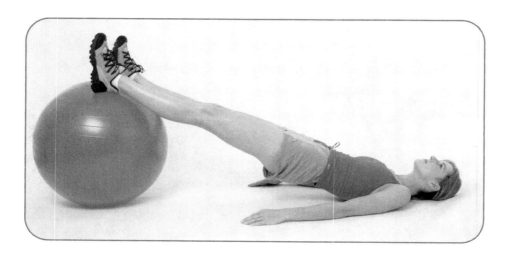

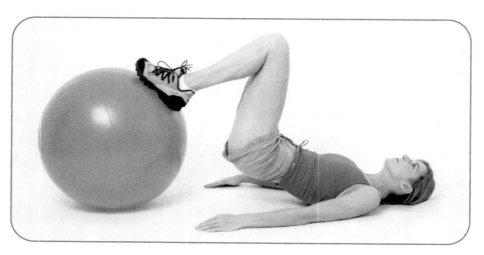

INNER-THIGH EXERCISE BALL SQUEEZE

Lie with your back flat on the floor. Place your hands behind your ears. With your legs in the air, slightly bent at the knee, place the ball in between your knees and your feet. Squeeze the ball for a few seconds as if you are trying to pop a balloon with your legs.

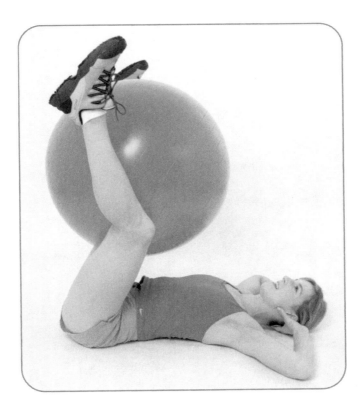

OUTER-THIGH HALF-MOON

Lie on your side on the floor. Rest your head and neck on your arm with your elbow on the floor. Bend your bottom leg at a 90-degree angle, keeping the top leg straight. Place the weight on the outer thigh of your top leg. Make sure your body is straight and your back is in alignment. Begin by lifting the leg straight up. In a half-moon motion, bring your leg forward, touching the floor with your toes. Again in a half-moon motion, bring your leg back up and back behind your bottom leg, touching the floor with your toes. Bring your leg back to center. Repeat on the other side.

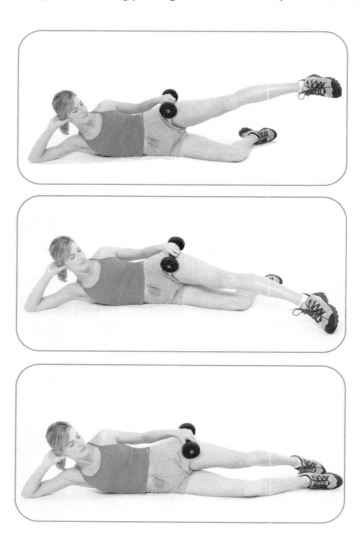

STANDING CALF RAISE

Place the weights in your hands, palms facing down. Keep arms straight alongside your body. Stand upright, feet facing forward. Lift straight up onto the balls of your feet. Squeeze your calf muscles, then slowly come back down to standing position.

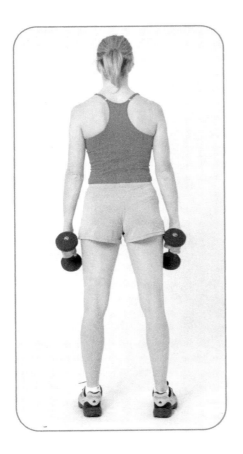
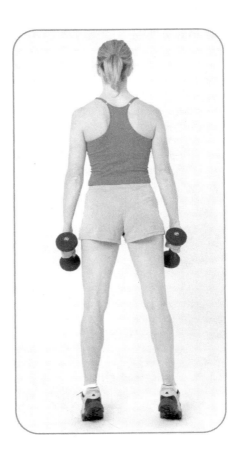

KNEE SWIMMER

Begin on your hands and knees. Knees should be hip width apart and hands should be shoulder width apart. Distribute your weight evenly. Back should be flat, head facing down toward the floor. Lift your leg straight, in alignment with your back. At the same time, bring the opposite arm straight out in front of you also in alignment with your back. Make sure to keep your belly tucked and your back straight. Repeat on the other side.

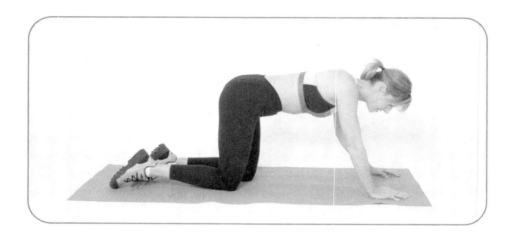

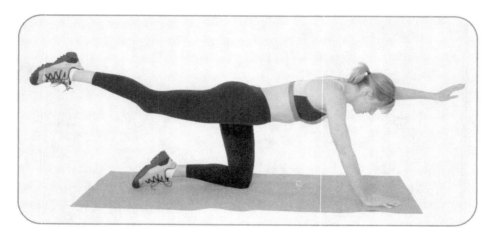

STANDING FRONT RAISE

Stand straight with feet slightly farther than hip width apart, knees relaxed. Place the weight in between your hands, palms facing inward. Begin with arms straight down in front of you, elbows slightly bent. Raise weight, keeping arms straight, to shoulder level. With control, bring weight back down to starting position.

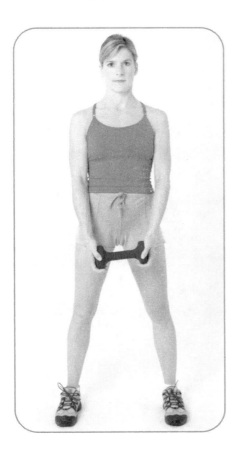 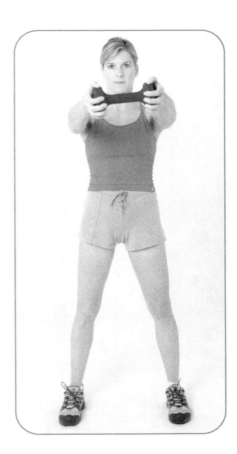

ONE-ARM EXERCISE BALL ROW

Place your knee and hand on the ball. Place your other leg next to the ball, keeping a slight bend in the knee. Keep your back straight by sticking out your butt and chest. Keep your head facing the ball. Begin by placing your outside arm straight down next to the ball. Bending your elbow, bring your arm straight up toward the ceiling. Squeeze your shoulder blade toward the middle of your body. Slowly bring your arm back down to starting position. Repeat on the other side.

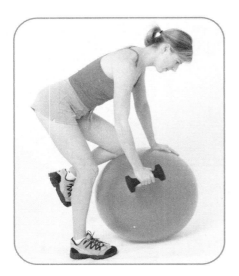 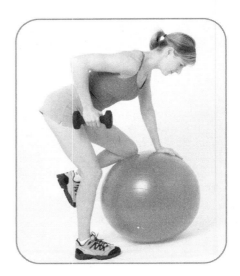

KNEE PUSH-UP

Place knees close together on the floor. Hands should be slightly farther than shoulder width apart. Keep your feet on the floor behind you, back straight. Begin upright with arms straight. Lower yourself so that your nose can almost touch the floor. Slowly bring yourself back to starting position.

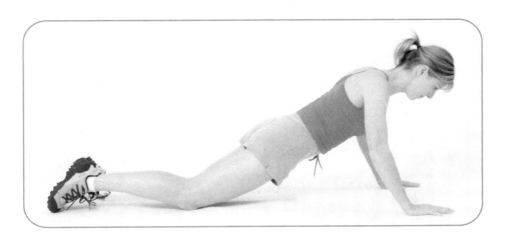

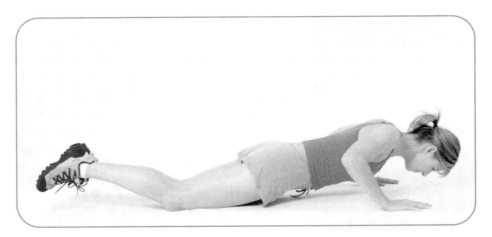

CHEST PRESS ON EXERCISE BALL

Lie with your upper back and neck on the ball. Create a table with your torso, bending your knees at a 90-degree angle directly above your feet. Push your hips up toward the ceiling to create a flat back. Keep this position throughout the exercise. Begin by holding the free weights, palms facing away from your head, elbows at 90 degrees. Push the free weights directly up toward the ceiling. Slowly bring them back down to starting position.

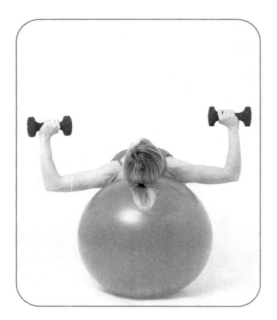 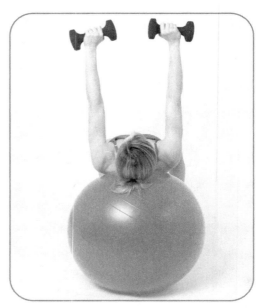

RESISTANCE-BAND PULL

Hold the resistance band in the center where you can feel enough tension, palms facing down. Begin by placing your arms out in front of you at chest level as if you have a big ball between your arms. Keep your elbows slightly bent throughout the exercise. Pull the exercise band apart, pulling your hands farther away from each other. Slowly bring them back to starting position.

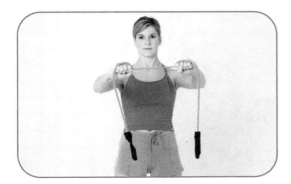 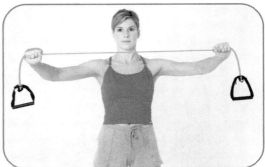

STANDING OVERHEAD PRESS WITH BAND

Hold the handles of the resistance band, palms facing inward. Step on the band so that you have an even amount of tubing on both sides. Begin with your arms at shoulder level, elbows at a 90-degree angle. Lift arms upward and inward toward the ceiling. Slowly bring arms back down to starting position. Make sure not to lower your arms past your shoulder level.

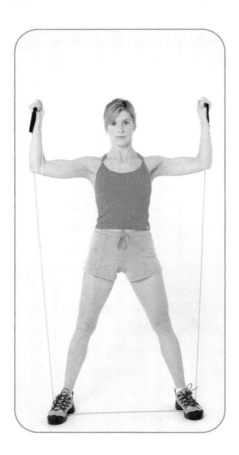 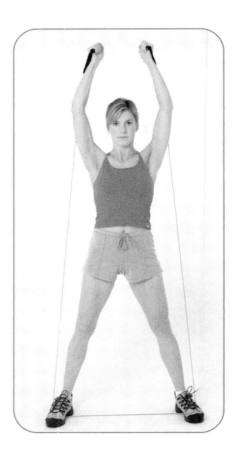

STANDING LATERAL RAISE

Stand straight with feet slightly farther than hip width apart, knees slightly bent. Place weights in hands, palms facing inward. Begin with your arms straight down at your sides, elbows slightly bent. Maintain that bend throughout the exercise. Lift arms straight out to shoulder level. Slowly bring your arms back down to starting position.

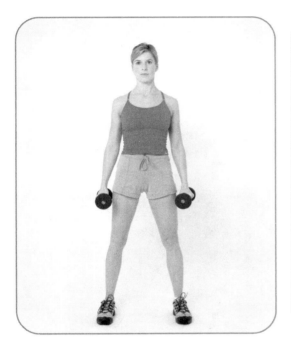 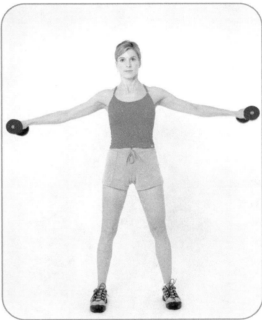

STANDING BICEPS CURL

Stand straight with feet slightly farther than hip width apart, knees slightly bent. Place the weights in your hands, palms facing forward. Begin with your arms straight down and slightly in front of your body. Keeping your elbows and upper arms at your sides, bring weights up toward the ceiling. Slowly bring arms back to starting position.

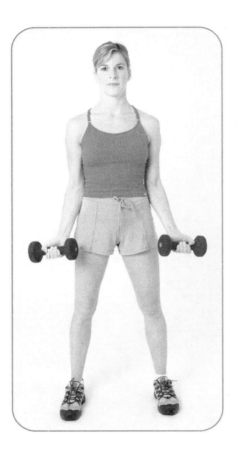 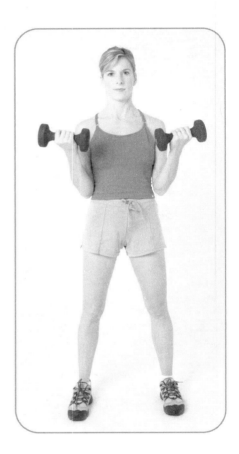

HAMMER CURL WITH BAND

Stand straight, holding the resistance band with palms facing inward. Step on the resistance band so that there is an even amount of tubing on each side. Begin with your arms straight down and slightly in front of your body. Keeping your elbows at your sides bring arms up toward the ceiling. Slowly bring arms back to starting position.

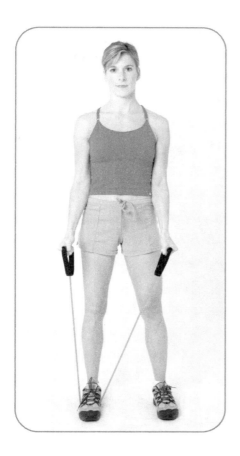 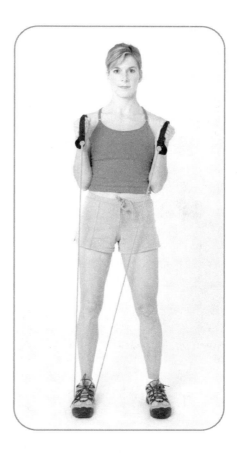

KNEE TRICEPS PUSH-UP

Place knees close together on the floor. Keep your feet on the floor behind you, back straight. Place your hands together creating a triangle by touching your thumbs and index fingers. Lower yourself to the ground to where your nose almost touches the floor. Slowly lift yourself back to starting position.

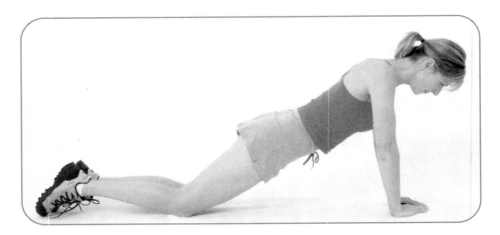

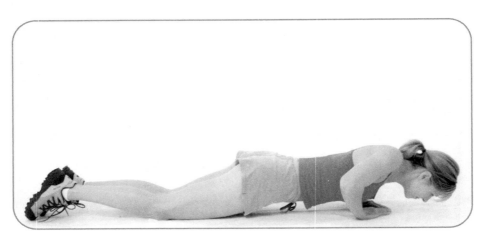

STANDING TRICEPS PRESS

Stand straight with feet slightly farther than hip width apart. Hold the weight directly over your head with both hands, palms toward the ceiling, thumbs interlaced. Begin with the weight directly over your head, elbows slightly bent. Lower weight behind you without moving your elbows. Slowly bring weight back to starting position.

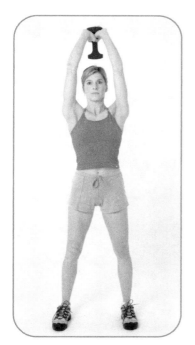
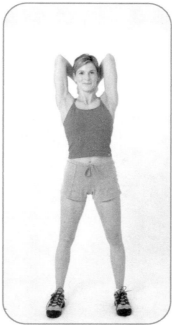
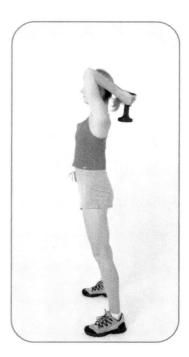

EXERCISE BALL CRUNCH ONE

Lie on the floor with your knees bent at a 90-degree angle and your heels on the ball. Place your hands behind your ears. Lift your shoulder blades off the floor, toward the ceiling. Keep your chin lifted and your arms out at the sides of your head throughout the exercise. You should not be able to see your elbows during this exercise. Slowly bring your body back to starting position.

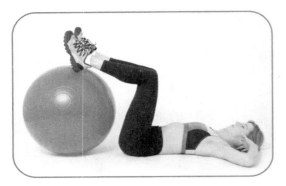 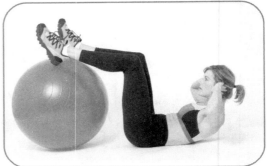

BIKE ON FLOOR

Lie on the floor with your hands on the back of your head. Lift your left shoulder blade up as you bring your right knee in toward your torso. Rotate your upper body so that your left elbow reaches toward your right knee. Repeat on the other side, never letting your feet touch the floor.

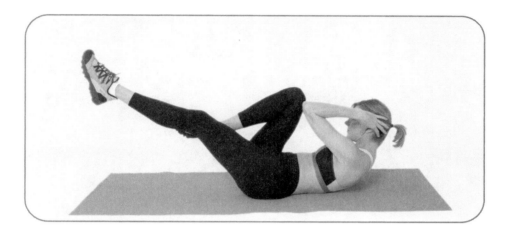

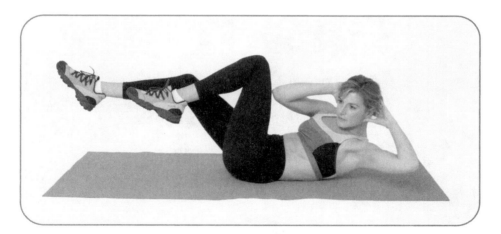

DEAD BUG

Lie on the floor with arms and legs extended toward the ceiling. Keep a 90-degree bend in your knees. Lower your opposite arm and leg, stopping a few inches above the floor. Bring arm and leg back to starting position. Repeat on the other side.

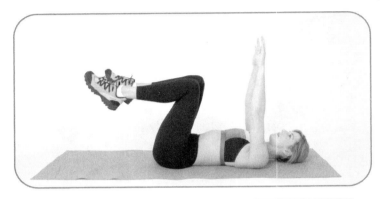

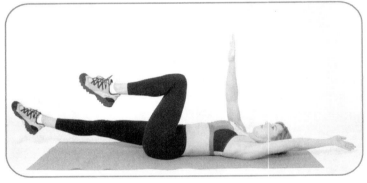

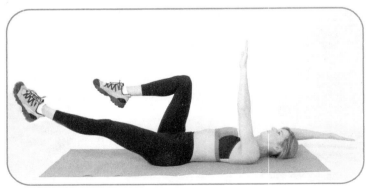

FLOOR OBLIQUE

Lie on your side on the floor, keeping your back straight. Begin by bringing your legs out in front of you, bending your knees slightly. Place your bottom arm straight out in front of you for balance. Do not push on your arm. Place your top hand on your ear. Lift your torso up and toward your hips, shortening your side abdominals. Slowly bring your torso back to starting position.

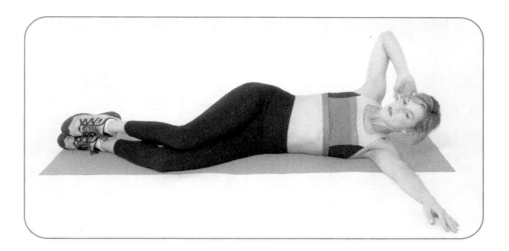

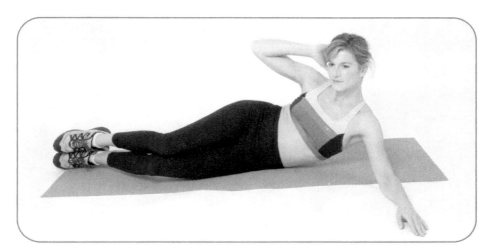

EXERCISE BALL PUSH-OUT

Begin on your knees with the heels of your hands pressed into the ball. Keeping your back straight, roll the ball away from you until your forearms are pressing into the ball. Slowly bring your body back to starting position.

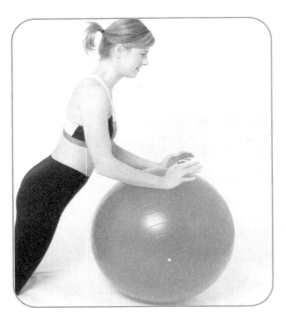 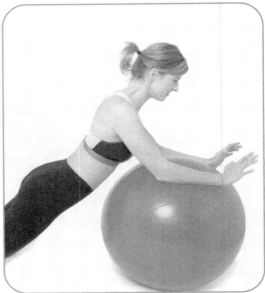

SIDE TOE TOUCH

Lie with your back flat on the floor, knees bent, feet on the floor hip width apart. Begin with your arms straight at your sides. Lift your shoulder blades off the floor, toward the ceiling. Rotate your upper body, trying to touch your fingers to your heel. Rotate your body to the other side, again trying to touch your fingers to your heel.

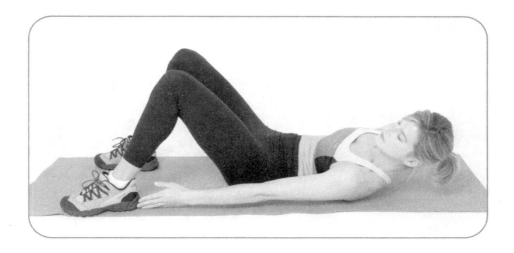

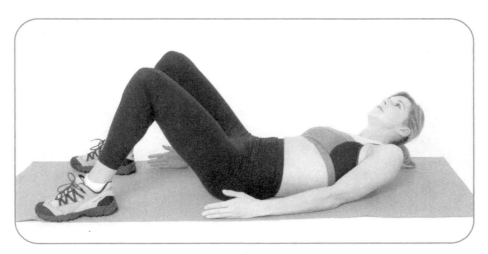

PLANK

Lie on the floor, facedown. Bring your elbows and forearms underneath your head. Your elbows should be directly under your shoulders. Lift your body off the ground, staying on your forearms and the toes of your feet. Keep your body straight. Hold as long as you can.

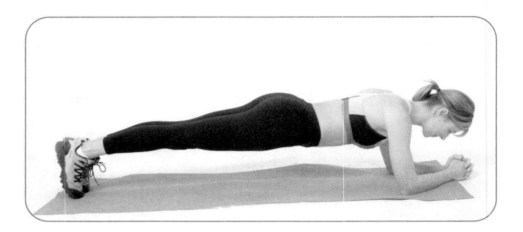

DOWNWARD DOG

Start on your hands, shoulder width apart, and on your knees, hip width apart. Lift up, making a V with your body and evenly distributing your weight on your hands and feet. Go deeper into the stretch by pushing your heels toward the floor and your butt toward the ceiling. Keep your back flat and your head relaxed. Hold for 30 seconds.

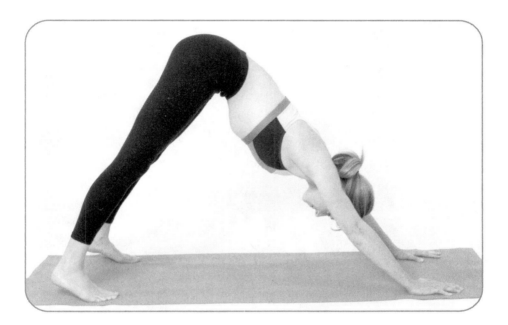

SPINAL TWIST

Sit on the floor, legs straight out in front of you. With your knee bent, bring your foot onto the other side of your leg. Keeping your back straight, bring your arm across your leg, resting your elbow against your thigh. Place your other arm behind you. Rotate your upper body toward your back arm. Hold for 30 seconds. Repeat on the other side.

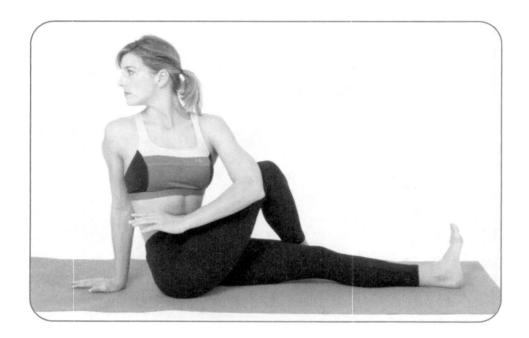

PIGEON

Begin in the downward-dog stretch. Bring your leg underneath you, knee bent. Align your knee with the center of your chest, your back leg straight out behind you. Sit with your upper body straight, arms at your sides for balance. Go deeper into the stretch by pushing your hips toward the floor and laying your upper body on the floor. Hold for 30 seconds. Repeat on the other side.

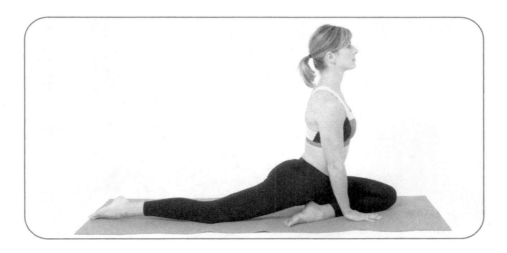

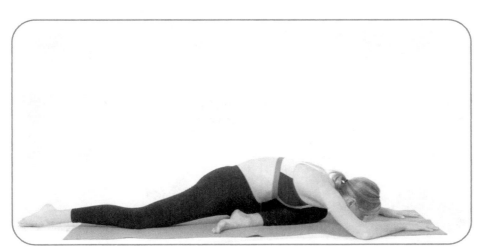

QUADRICEPS STRETCH

Begin in the pigeon stretch. Lift the lower part of your back leg off the ground, holding it with your hand. Push your hips into the ground to go deeper into the stretch. Hold for 30 seconds. Repeat on the other side.

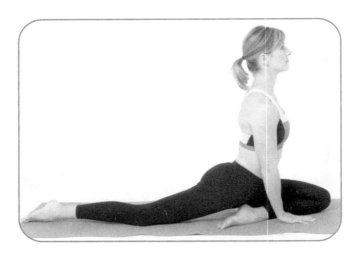

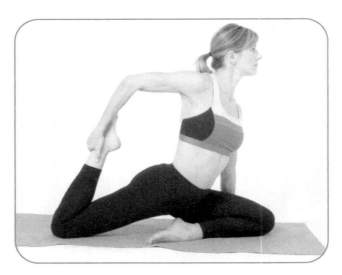

HAMSTRING STRETCH

Sit on the ground with legs straight out in front of you. Bending at the hips, bring your torso to your thighs. If you can't reach your toes, use a resistance band to help push you deeper into the stretch. If you can reach your feet, wrap your index and middle fingers around your big toes to help push you deeper into the stretch. Hold for 30 seconds.

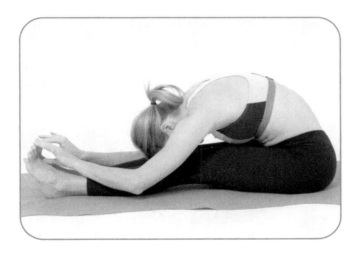

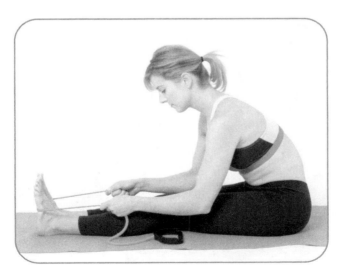

CALF STRETCH

Lie on your back with your leg straight in the air, foot flexed. Place the resistance band on the ball of your foot and pull your foot down toward you. Hold for a few seconds, then rotate your ankle inward so that the bottom of your foot is facing inward. Hold for 30 seconds. Repeat on the other side.

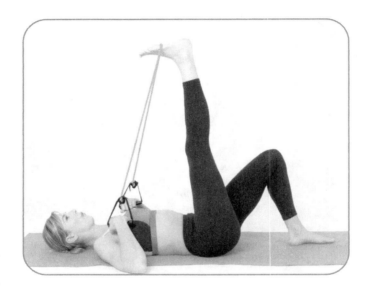

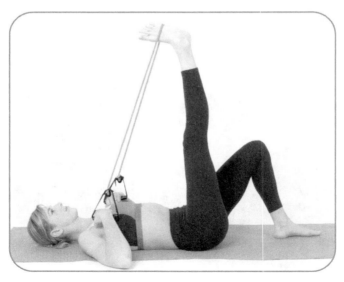

CHEST AND BICEPS STRETCH

Stand arm's length away from the wall. Place your left arm against the wall, thumb facing the ceiling. Keeping your shoulder relaxed, twist away from the wall. Hold for 30 seconds. Repeat on the other side.

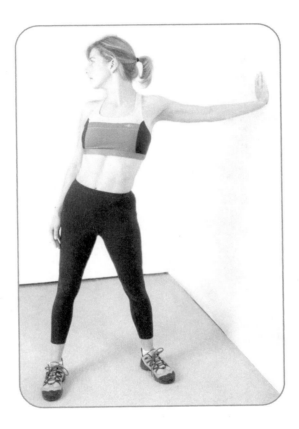

SHOULDER STRETCH

Standing straight, bring one arm behind you so that your hand is between your shoulder blades. Bend your other arm, trying to grab your bottom hand with your top hand. If you can't reach, use a resistance band to push yourself deeper into the stretch. If you can reach, grasp your hands and pull to go deeper into the stretch. Hold for 30 seconds. Gently let go. Repeat on the other side.

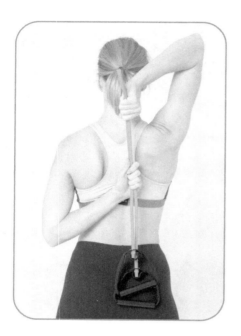 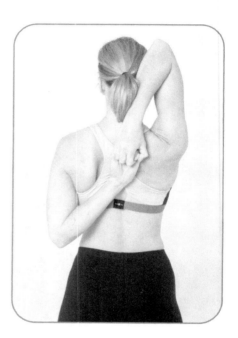

TRICEPS STRETCH

Standing straight, bring one arm up, bending at the elbow. With your other arm, grab just below your elbow. Pull your arm inward with your opposite hand to go deeper into the stretch. Hold for 30 seconds. Repeat on the other side.

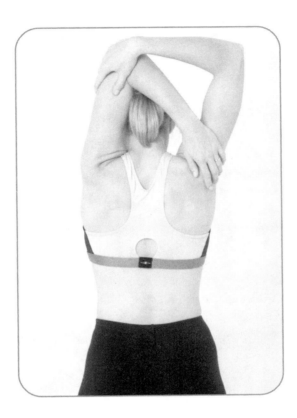

ADVANCED

Congratulations! You have just graduated to Advanced. There's no retreating now! At this time you're probably completing the guest list, ordering the invitations, and deciding on your wedding cake. Your big day is just a few months away and you are energized, getting stronger, losing weight, and trimming down. No time for complacency now. It's time to shake it up and challenge the body again.

At this stage you are going to choose some new exercises and kick up the intensity. If you've been walking, it's time to add running intervals (walk ten minutes, run two minutes, walk ten minutes, run two minutes). Maintain a four-day cardio plan. If you've been doing kickboxing classes, then try something new. Are the seasons changing? Take up surfing, volleyball, snowboarding, or cross-country skiing. Each is a fantastic and fun workout.

Instead of doing Basic two times a week, you will be doing Advanced. As with Basic, your goal is to perform thirty repetitions of each exercise, moving to the next without a break. Advanced is more difficult, so don't worry if you actually have to decrease your weights for the first couple of weeks. You will also be doing a few core exercises for posture and a trim torso. A strong core leads to a tall, lean body and will ensure that you are standing tall and looking terrific on your wedding day.

Your aerobic routine should also get a little bit harder, continuing to challenge your body so that you don't plateau.

For your flexibility training in this level, refer back to the Basic program flexibility guidelines. Even though the stretches themselves have not changed, you will probably notice that you are more limber and can stretch farther than when you began. Gently and safely push yourself to stretch deeper each time.

Real Brides: Tips from the Trenches

Good posture can take ten pounds off your body through the camera lens. So work those abs and stand tall on your wedding day. Slouching is never attractive. For your formal wedding photos don't forget to hold your arms out, slightly away from your body. This little photographer's trick will make your upper body look even more trim and your arms seem extremely toned.

EXERCISE	MUSCLE GROUP
Warm-up	5 minutes: treadmill, bike, or jumping rope
Stretch	2 minutes: all major muscle groups
Backward Lunge with Knee Lift	Legs
Plié Squat with Skier Lift	Legs
Hamstring Roll on Elbows	Legs
Inner-Thigh Exercise Ball Squeeze	Legs
Outer-Thigh Half-Moon	Legs
Standing Angled Calf Raise	Legs
Swimmer on Ball	Back
Seated Front Raise	Back
Bent-Over Row	Back
One-Arm Exercise Ball Chest Press	Chest
Straight Push-up off Ball	Chest
Standing Overhead Press with Band	Shoulder
Seated Lateral Raise	Shoulder
Seated Biceps Curl	Biceps
Hammer Curl with Band	Biceps
Straight Triceps Push-up	Triceps
Seated Triceps Push-Down	Triceps
Exercise Ball Crunch Two	Abdominals
Bike on Ball	Abdominals
Kayaker	Abdominals
Oblique with Leg Lifts	Abdominals
Stick Crunch	Abdominals
Extended Crunch	Abdominals
Ball Balance	Core
Rotating Plank	Core
Downward Dog	Flexibility
Spinal Twist	Flexibility
Pigeon	Flexibility
Quadriceps Stretch	Flexibility
Hamstring Stretch	Flexibility
Calf Stretch	Flexibility
Chest and Biceps Stretch	Flexibility
Shoulder Stretch	Flexibility
Triceps Stretch	Flexibility

BACKWARD LUNGE WITH KNEE LIFT

Stand straight with both feet facing forward, arms holding weights at your side. Keeping your upper body straight, place your leg straight behind you, far enough back to perform a lunge. Dip straight down, bending both knees. Do not let your front knee go beyond your ankle. Lift straight up, bringing your leg up in front of you, knee bent. Slowly bring your leg back to starting position. Repeat on other side.

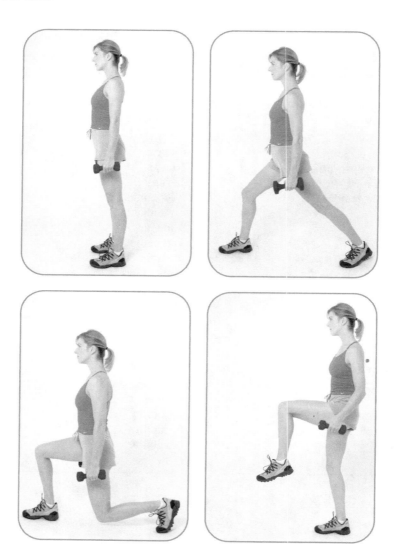

PLIÉ SQUAT WITH SKIER LIFT

Stand straight with legs wider than hip width apart. Bring your arms in front of you at chest level for balance. Squat down, sticking out your butt as if you are trying to sit down. Bring your body back up to starting position, bringing your leg straight out to the side. Bring your leg back down, repeat the squat, then repeat with the leg lift on the other side.

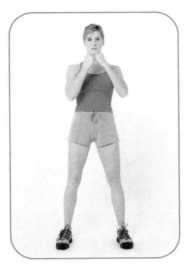
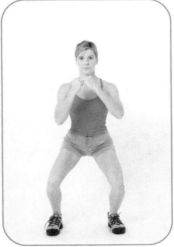
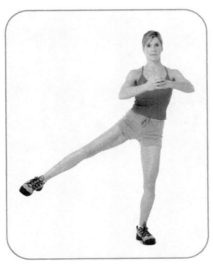

HAMSTRING ROLL ON ELBOWS

Lie flat on the floor with the heels of your feet on the ball and your arms at your sides, close to your body, forearms off the ground. To begin, lift your torso off the floor creating a straight plank with your body. Using your hamstring and calf muscles, pull the ball toward you, keeping your upper body straight. Slowly bring the ball back to starting position.

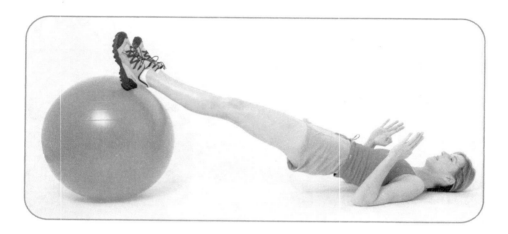

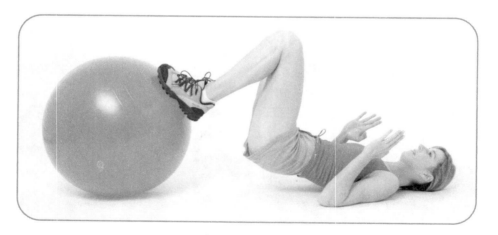

INNER-THIGH EXERCISE BALL SQUEEZE

Lie with your back flat on the floor. Place your hands by your head. With your legs straight up in the air and knees slightly bent, place the ball in between your knees and your feet. Keep your legs and the ball in this position throughout the exercise. To perform the exercise, squeeze the ball for a few seconds as if you are trying to pop a balloon with your legs.

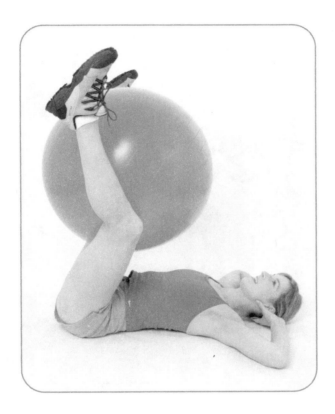

OUTER-THIGH HALF-MOON

Lie on your side on the floor. Rest your head and neck on your arm with your elbow on the floor. Bend your bottom leg at a 90-degree angle, keeping the top leg straight. Place the weight on the outer thigh of your top leg. Make sure your body is straight and your back is in alignment. Begin by lifting the leg straight up. In a half-moon motion, bring your leg forward, touching the floor with your toes. Again in a half-moon motion, bring your leg back up and back behind your bottom leg, touching the floor with your toes. Bring your leg back to center. Repeat on the other side.

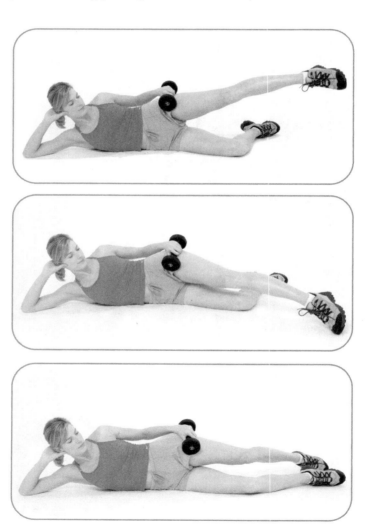

STANDING ANGLED CALF RAISE

Place weights in your hands, palms facing inward. Keep arms straight directly alongside your body. To begin, stand upright, toes facing outward. Lift straight up onto the balls of your feet. Squeeze your calf muscles, then slowly come back down to standing position.

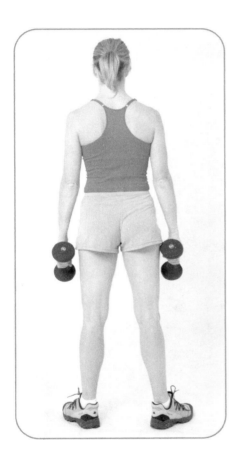 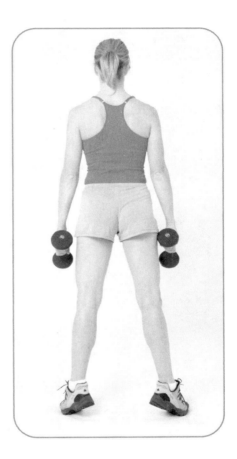

SWIMMER ON BALL

Lie face forward with your torso on the ball. Extend your legs straight behind you with the balls of your feet on the floor. Place both hands on the floor in front of the ball. Begin by lifting one leg and the opposite arm off the floor, creating a straight line with your body. Slowly bring them back down to the floor and repeat on the other side.

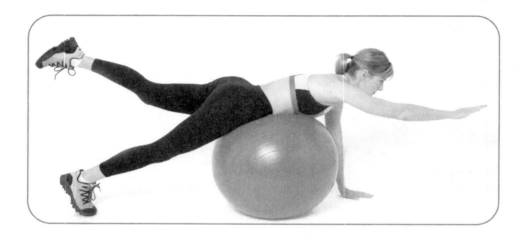

SEATED FRONT RAISE

Sit upright on the ball with your legs in front of you. Place the weight in your hands, palms facing inward. Begin with arms extended toward your thighs, elbows slightly bent. Maintaining your balance on the ball, raise weight to shoulder level, keeping arms straight. Slowly bring weight back down to starting position.

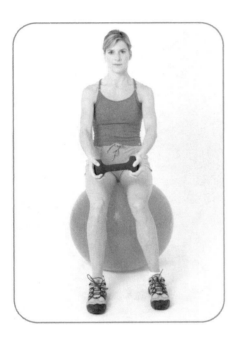 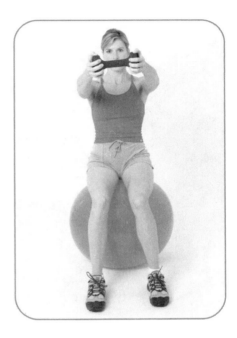

BENT-OVER ROW

Stand with your legs together, bent over at the hips. Keep your back straight by sticking out your butt and your chest. Begin with your arms straight down at your sides, elbows slightly bent. Lift your arms up to shoulder level. Slowly bring your arms back to starting position.

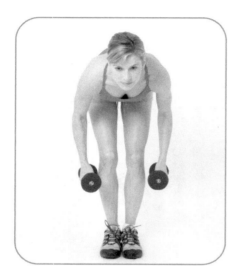 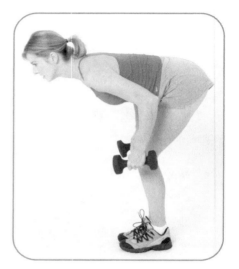

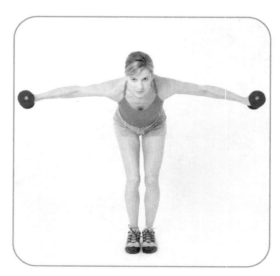

ONE-ARM EXERCISE BALL CHEST PRESS

Lie with your upper back and neck on the ball. Create a table with your torso, bending your knees at a 90-degree angle directly above your feet. Push your hips up toward the ceiling to create a flat back. Keep this position throughout the exercise. Begin by holding the weights, palms facing away from your head, elbows at 90 degrees. Lift one arm straight to the ceiling. With control, bring the arm back down to starting position. Repeat on the other side.

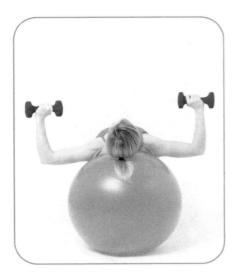 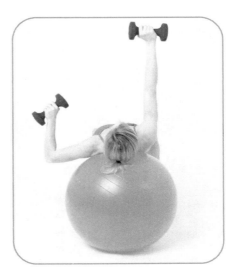

STRAIGHT PUSH-UP OFF BALL

Place the tops of your feet on top of the ball. Keeping your back straight, place your arms slightly wider than shoulder width apart. Lower yourself so that your nose can almost touch the floor. Slowly bring yourself back to starting position.

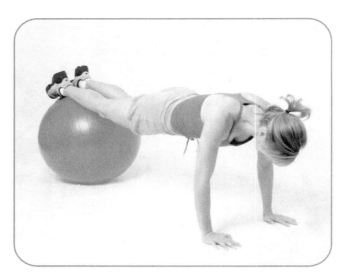

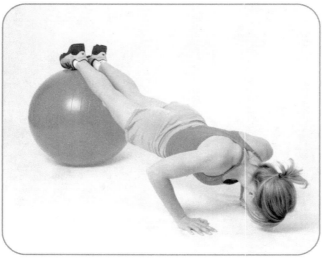

STANDING OVERHEAD PRESS WITH BAND

Hold the handles of the resistance band, palms facing inward. Step on the band so that you have an even amount of tubing on both sides. Begin with your arms at shoulder level, elbows at a 90-degree angle. Lift arms upward and inward toward the ceiling. Slowly bring arms back down to starting position. Make sure not to lower your arms past your shoulder level.

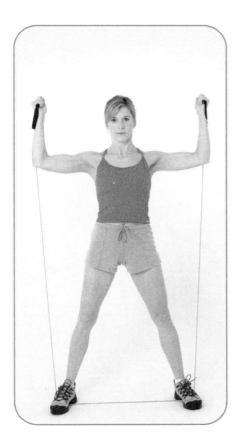 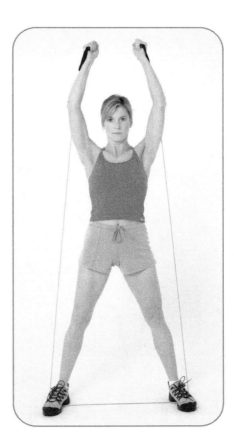

SEATED LATERAL RAISE

Sit upright on the ball with your legs in front of you. Place the weights in your hands, palms facing inward. Begin with your arms extended down at your sides, elbows slightly bent. Maintaining your balance on the ball, raise weights to the sides, keeping arms straight, to shoulder level. Slowly bring your arms back to the starting position.

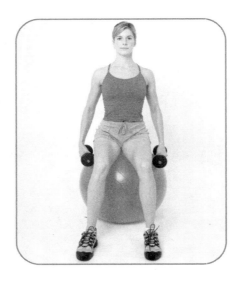

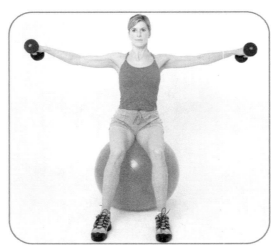

SEATED BICEPS CURL

Sit upright on the ball with your legs in front of you. Place the weights in your hands, palms facing forward. Begin with your arms straight down at your sides. Keeping your elbows and upper arms at your sides, bring weights up toward the ceiling. Slowly bring arms back to starting position.

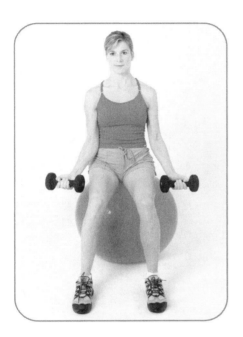 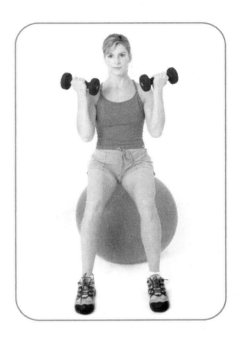

HAMMER CURL WITH BAND

Stand straight, holding the resistance band with palms facing inward. Step on the resistance band so that there is an even amount of tubing on each side. Begin with your arms straight down and slightly in front of your body. Keeping your elbows and upper arms at your sides, bring arms up toward the ceiling. Slowly bring arms back to starting position.

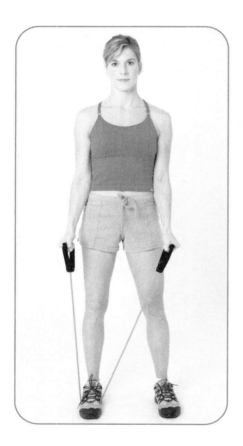 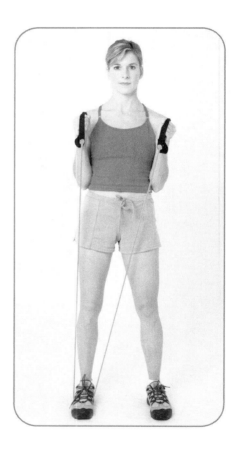

STRAIGHT TRICEPS PUSH-UP

Place knees close together on the floor. Lift up onto the balls of your feet, keeping your back straight. Place your hands together creating a triangle by touching your thumbs and index fingers. Lower yourself to where your nose almost touches the floor. Slowly lift yourself back to starting position.

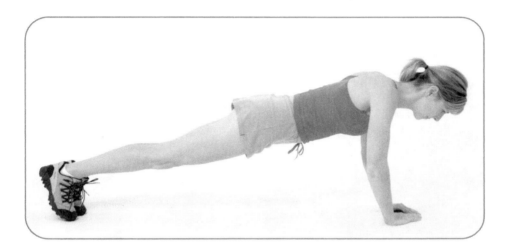

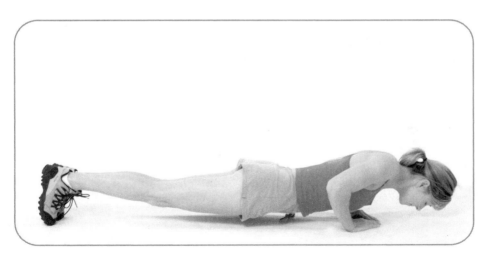

SEATED TRICEPS PUSH-DOWN

Sit upright on the ball with your legs in front of you. Hold the weight directly over your head with both hands, palms toward the ceiling, thumbs interlaced. Begin with the weight directly over your head, elbows slightly bent. Lower weight behind you until your elbows are at a 90-degree angle. Slowly bring weight back to starting position.

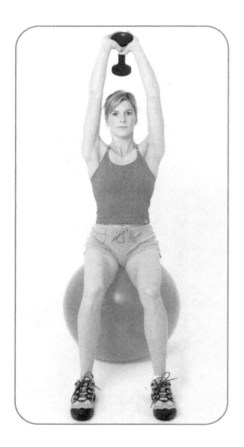 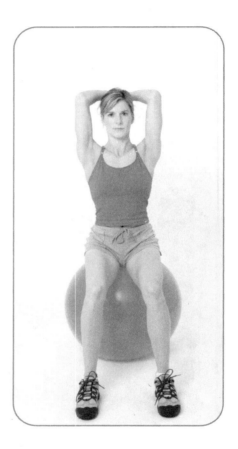

EXERCISE BALL CRUNCH TWO

Sit on the ball with your legs out in front of you. Place your hands behind your ears. Lie on the ball so that your torso is extended. Lift your torso up and forward, stopping when only your butt and lower back are still on the ball. Slowly bring your body back to starting position.

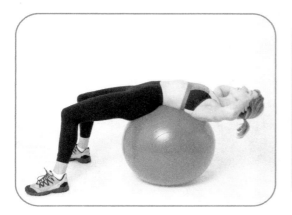 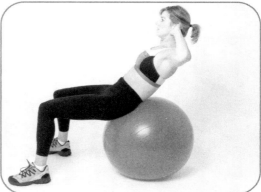

BIKE ON BALL

Lie on the floor with the heels of your feet on the ball. Place your hands behind your ears. Lift your shoulder blades off the floor. Bring one knee toward your chest and rotate your upper body, bringing your opposite elbow to your knee. Repeat on the other side.

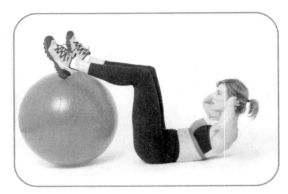

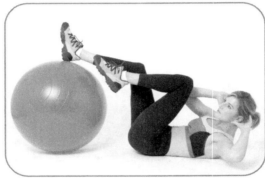

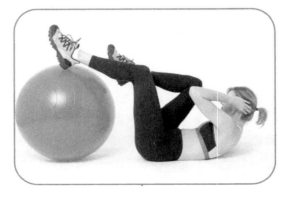

KAYAKER

Create a V with your body by placing your feet together on the floor and leaning back with your upper body. Place a weight in your hands, palms facing inward. Keep the weight at waist level. Touch the weight on the floor side to side by rotating your torso.

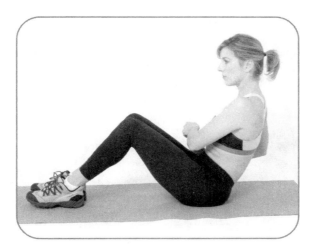

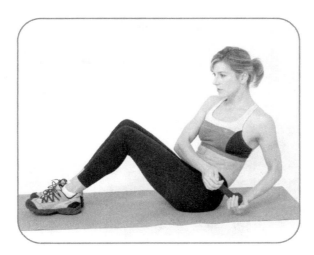

OBLIQUE WITH LEG LIFTS

Lie on your side on the floor, keeping your back straight. Bring your legs out in front of you slightly, bending your knees. Place your bottom arm straight out in front of you for balance. Do not push on your arm. Place your top hand on your ear. Lift your torso up and down toward your hips. At the same time, bring your legs off the floor and bring your knees toward your chest. Slowly bring your legs and torso back down without letting them touch the floor. Repeat on the other side.

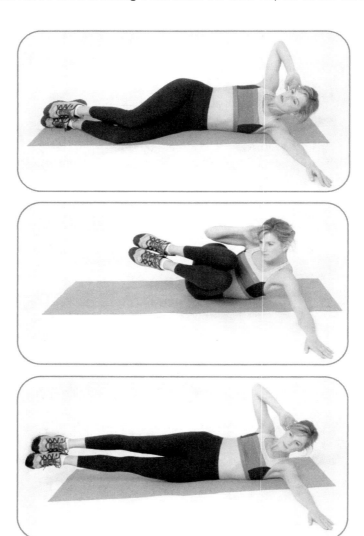

STICK CRUNCH

Lie on the floor with your legs up in the air, knees bent at a 90-degree angle. Place a weight in your hands, palms facing inward. Begin with your arms up in the air, elbows bent at a 90-degree angle. Bring your lower body up and toward your arms. At the same time, bring your arms toward your feet. Slowly bring your arms and legs back to starting position.

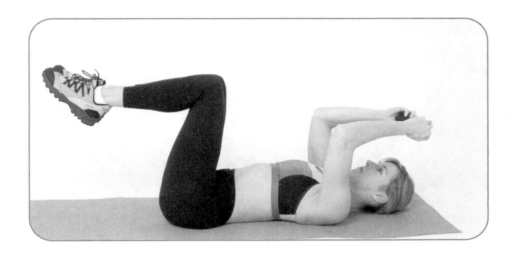

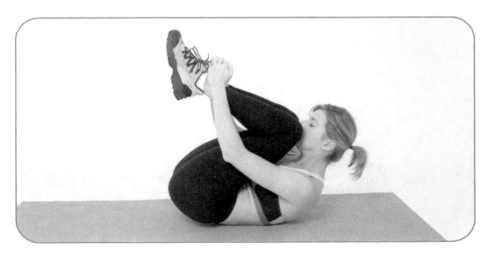

EXTENDED CRUNCH

Lie on the floor, back straight. Place your hands behind your ears. Set one foot on top of the other. Lift your shoulder blades off the floor up toward the ceiling. Keep your elbows out toward your sides. You should not be able to see your elbows. Slowly bring your shoulder blades back to starting position. Repeat, switching your feet.

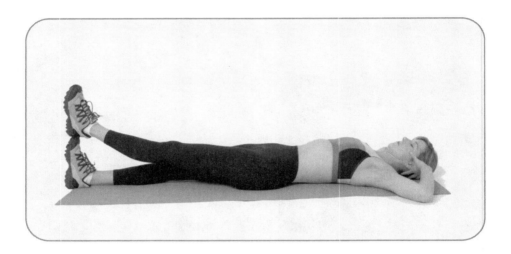

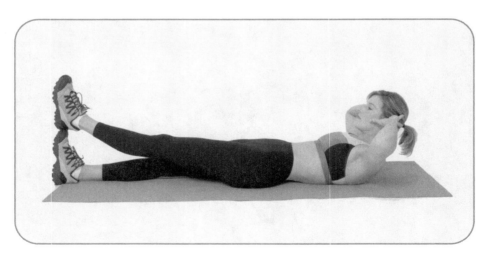

BALL BALANCE

Lie with your upper back and neck on the ball. Create a table with your torso, bending your knees at a 90-degree angle directly above your ankles. Push your hips up toward the ceiling to create a flat back. Keep this position throughout the exercise. Hold on to the ball with your hands. Slowly lift one leg off the ground and extend it out in front of you. With control, bring the leg back to starting position. Repeat on the other side.

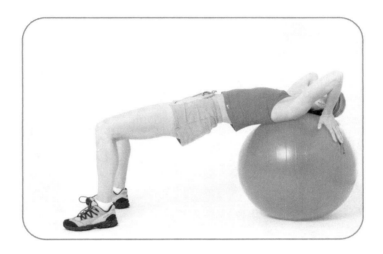

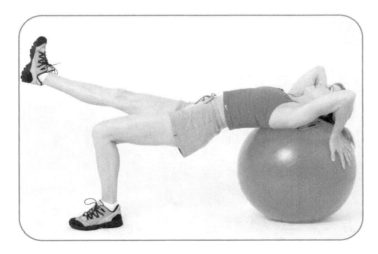

ROTATING PLANK

Start in a straight push-up position, legs close together and hands shoulder width apart on the floor. Maintain a straight torso and hips throughout the exercise. Rotate to one side, keeping one arm underneath you as the other arm extends toward the ceiling. Hold for a few seconds. Slowly bring your body back to starting position, then repeat on the other side.

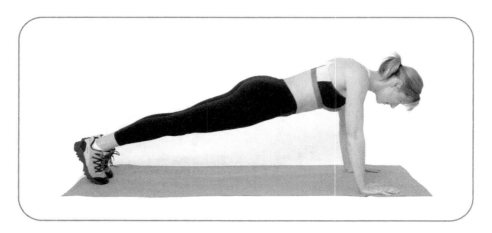

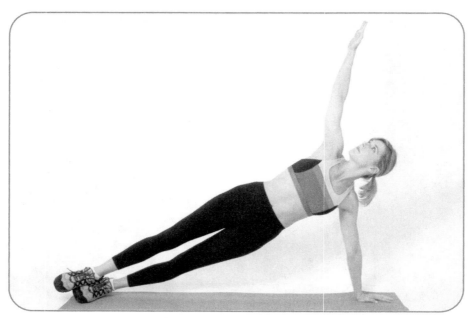

HARD CORE

Congratulations! You've reached another milestone on your road to fitness! The invitations are in the mail, the wedding rings have been purchased, and the honeymoon is booked. You've started to attend bridal showers and to shop for guest favors and attendant gifts. The wedding is fast approaching and you've come a long way, soldier, so don't lose focus now!

You've kicked it up a notch and are still moving forward. This is the high-intensity stage. No turning back now! We are upping the intensity by adding more high-impact aerobic workouts, four to five days a week. You know the drill, choose two new exercises and get moving. At this point, feel free to add another day and mix up your aerobic workouts by doing more than one exercise in a workout session. I like to combine running and biking, doing thirty to forty minutes of each. Pick high-intensity exercises that are going to make you sweat. You know you can do it!

Try exercises that were once out of reach. You won't know if you can do them unless you give it a shot.

The Hard Core strength-training routine will be even more challenging and includes extra arm and back exercises for that sleeveless, strapless, or even backless wedding dress you will be wearing. Continue to be diligent about doing your flexibility exercises. It will pay off in the end.

At this point you have trimmed down and toned up. Continue to dedicate two days a week to your strength training. Feeling slim and focused on building muscle? Add a third day of full-body Hard Core strength training to your week.

You are now skilled in the Bootcamp360 strength-training philosophy. Work toward thirty repetitions and keep moving quickly from one exercise to the next.

> **Your body is your best accessory. Remember, it is you that makes the dress look great—not the other way around.**

EXERCISE	MUSCLE GROUP
Warm-up	5 minutes: treadmill, bike, or jumping rope
Stretch	2 minutes: all major muscle groups
Backward Lunge with Punches	Legs
Squat Kicks	Legs
Hamstring Roll, No Arms	Legs
Inner-Thigh Lift	Legs
Outer-Thigh Half-Moon	Legs
Standing Angled Calf Raise	Legs
Lift and Rotate	Back
Seated Leg-Lifted Front Raise	Back
Overhead Raise on Ball	Back
Wide Row on Ball	Back
Push-up on Ball	Chest
Chest Fly on Ball	Chest
Standing Overhead Press with Band	Shoulder
Seated Leg-Lifted Lateral Raise	Shoulder
Seated Leg-Lifted Biceps Curl	Biceps
Hammer Curl with Band	Biceps
Triceps Push-Down	Triceps
Triceps Dip off Ball	Triceps
Kickback on Ball	Triceps
Exercise Ball Crunch Three	Abdominals
Bike on Ball	Abdominals
Oblique on Ball	Abdominals
Rolling Jackknife	Abdominals
Kayaker with Legs	Abdominals
Rotating Plank	Abdominals
Downward Dog	Flexibility
Spinal Twist	Flexibility
Pigeon	Flexibility
Quadriceps Stretch	Flexibility
Hamstring Stretch	Flexibility
Calf Stretch	Flexibility
Chest and Biceps Stretch	Flexibility
Shoulder Stretch	Flexibility
Triceps Stretch	Flexibility

BACKWARD LUNGE WITH PUNCHES

Stand straight with both feet facing forward, arms down holding weights. Keeping your upper body straight, place one leg straight behind you, far enough back to perform a lunge. Dip straight down, bending both knees. Do not let your front knee go beyond your ankle. At the same time punch forward with the arm opposite the forward knee. Lift straight up, bringing your back leg up in front of you, knee bent, punching with the other arm. Slowly bring your leg back to starting position. Repeat on the other side.

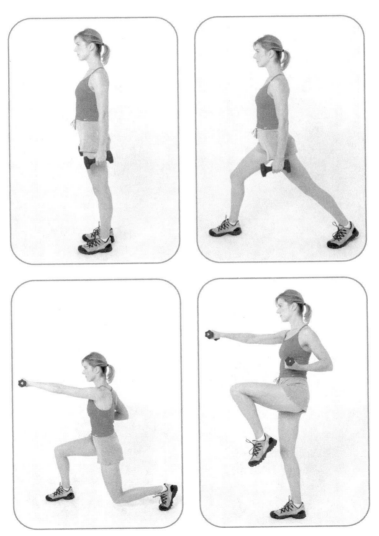

SQUAT KICKS

Stand straight with legs wider than hip width apart, feet facing forward. Squat down, sticking your butt out as if you are trying to sit down. Lift yourself upright, bringing your knee up, kicking forward. Bring your leg back to starting position, repeat the squat, and kick the same leg to the side. Bring your leg back to the starting position, repeat the squat, and kick the same leg back. Keep your back straight throughout the exercise. Repeat on the other side.

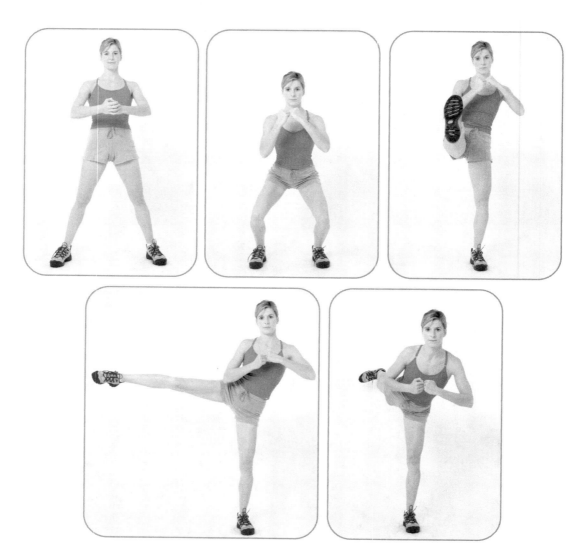

HAMSTRING ROLL, NO ARMS

Lie flat on the floor with the heels of your feet on top of the ball and arms crossed on your chest. To begin, lift your torso off the floor creating a straight plank with your body. Using your hamstring and calf muscles, pull the ball toward you, keeping your upper body straight. Slowly bring the ball back to its original position.

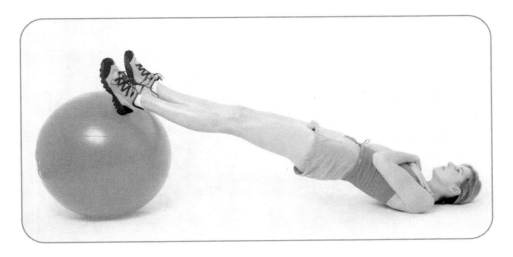

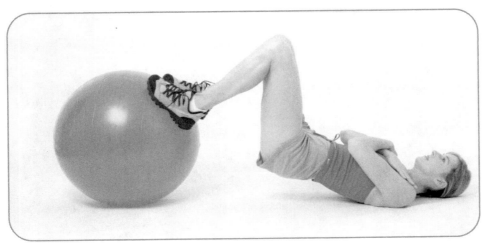

INNER-THIGH LIFT

Lie on your side on the floor. Place the weight of your upper body on your forearm. Bend your top leg, placing your foot on the floor behind your bottom leg. Place the weight on your inner thigh, keeping it in place with your hand. Keeping your leg straight, lift it toward the ceiling, foot flexed. Slowly bring your leg back down to starting position. Repeat on the other side.

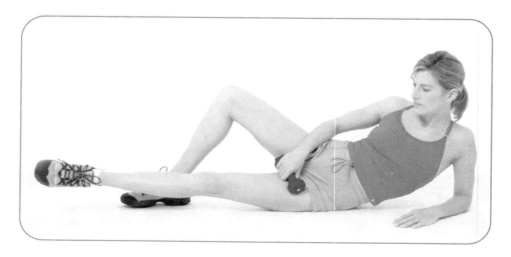

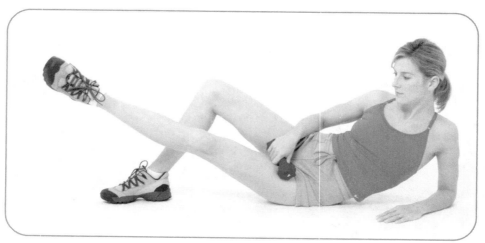

OUTER-THIGH HALF-MOON

Lie on your side on the floor. Rest your head and neck on your arm with your elbow on the floor. Bend your bottom leg at a 90-degree angle, keeping the top leg straight. Place the weight on the outer thigh of your top leg. Make sure your body is straight and your back in alignment. Begin by lifting the leg straight up. In a half-moon motion, bring your leg forward, touching the floor with your toes. Again in a half-moon motion, bring your leg back up and back behind your bottom leg, touching the floor with your toes. Bring your leg back to center. Repeat on the other side.

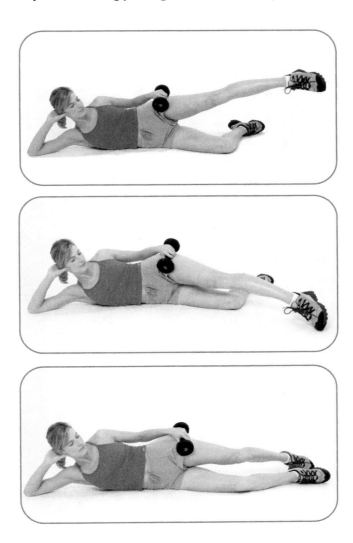

STANDING ANGLED CALF RAISE

Place weights in your hands, palms facing down. Keep arms straight directly alongside your body. To begin, stand upright, toes facing outward. Lift straight up onto the balls of your feet. Squeeze your calf muscles, then slowly come back down to standing position.

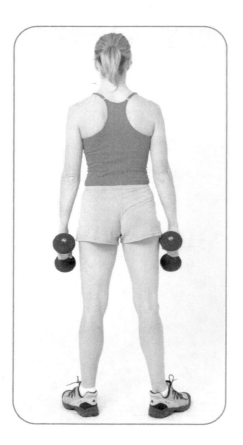 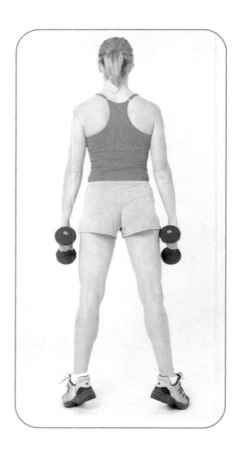

LIFT AND ROTATE

Lie with your torso on the ball and your feet securely against the wall. Place your hands behind your ears, elbows out. You should not be able to see your elbows. Begin extended over the ball. Lift up and then slowly bring yourself back down. Lift your torso up again, rotating to one side, and then slowly bring yourself back down. Lift and rotate to the other side.

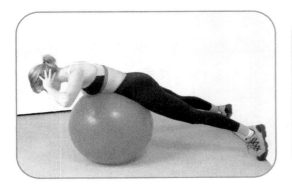

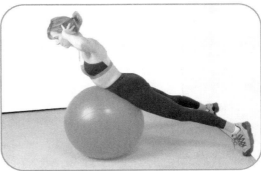

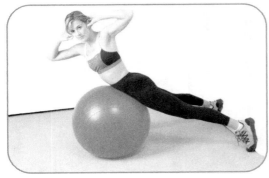

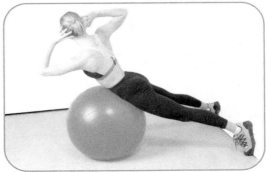

SEATED LEG-LIFTED FRONT RAISE

Sit upright on the ball with your legs in front of you. Place the weight in your hands, palms facing inward. Lift one leg off the floor a few inches. Begin with arms straight toward your thighs, elbows slightly bent. Keeping your balance, lift the weight in front of you to shoulder level. Slowly bring the weight back down to starting position, keeping the leg lifted.

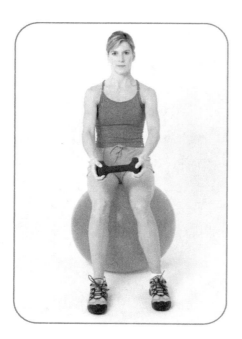 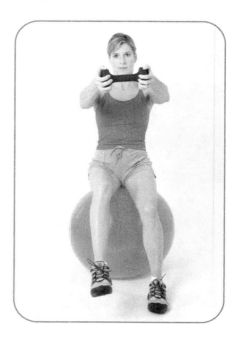

OVERHEAD RAISE ON BALL

Lie with your upper back and neck on the ball. Create a table with your torso, bending your knees at a 90-degree angle directly above your feet. Push your hips up toward the ceiling to create a flat back. Keep this position throughout the exercise. Place the weight in your hands, palms facing inward. Begin with your arms extended to the ceiling, maintaining a small bend in your elbows throughout the exercise. With extended arms, move the weight over your head until it is parallel with your body. Slowly bring the weight back to starting position.

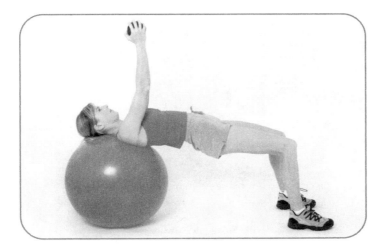

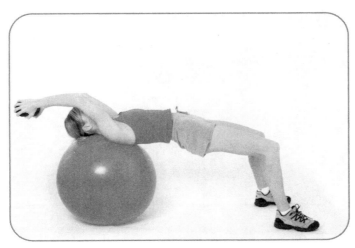

WIDE ROW ON BALL

Lie with your torso and chest on the ball. Extend your legs straight out behind you with the toes of your feet on the floor. With the weights in your hands, begin with your arms straight down on the floor on the sides of the ball. Lift your arms on the sides to shoulder level, squeezing your shoulder blades together. With control, bring your arms back to starting position.

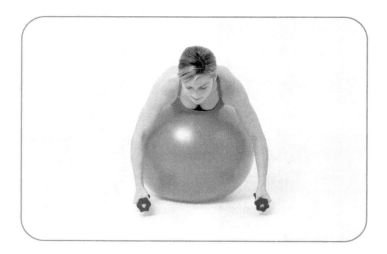

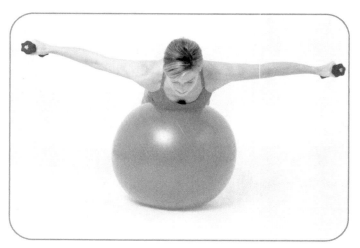

PUSH-UP ON BALL

Get into push-up position by placing your hands on the ball and your feet hip width apart on the floor, balanced against a wall. Straighten out your back, making a plank with your body. Begin with your arms straight and lower yourself closer to the ball until your chest almost touches the ball. Slowly lift yourself back to starting position.

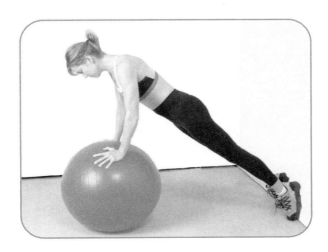

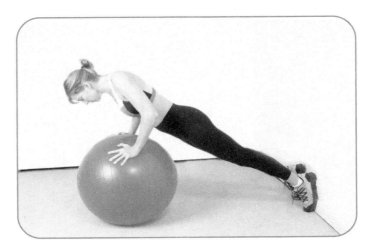

CHEST FLY ON BALL

Lie with your upper back and neck on the ball. Create a table with your torso, bending your knees at a 90-degree angle directly above your feet. Push your hips up toward the ceiling to create a flat back. Keep this position throughout the exercise. Begin by holding the weights in your hands, palms facing away from your face. Hands should be in alignment with your elbows. Lift the weights toward the ceiling as if there were a large ball on your chest, bringing your arms wide and up toward the ceiling. Slowly bring the weights back down to starting position.

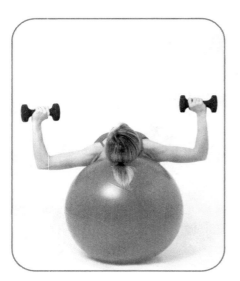 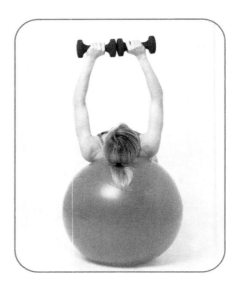

STANDING OVERHEAD PRESS WITH BAND

Hold the handles of the resistance band, palms facing inward. Step on the band so that you have an even amount of tubing on both sides. Begin with your arms at shoulder level, elbows at a 90-degree angle. Lift arms upward and inward toward the ceiling. Slowly bring arms back down to starting position. Make sure not to lower your arms past your shoulder level.

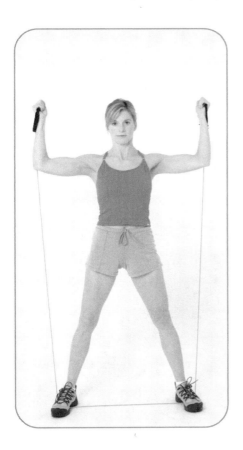
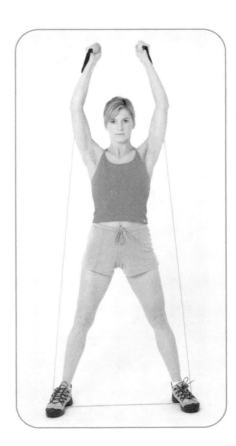

SEATED LEG-LIFTED LATERAL RAISE

Sit upright on the ball with your legs in front of you. Place the weights in your hands, palms facing inward. Lift your leg off the floor a few inches. Begin with your arms extended down at your sides, elbows slightly bent. Raise your arms to shoulder level. Slowly bring your arms back to starting position, keeping your leg lifted.

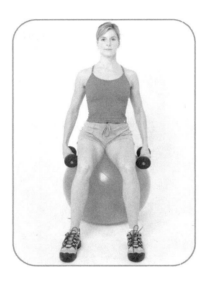

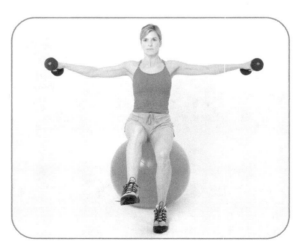

SEATED LEG-LIFTED BICEPS CURL

Sit upright on the ball with your legs out in front of you. Place the weights in your hands, palms facing forward. Lift your leg off the floor a few inches. Begin with your arms straight down at your sides. Keeping your elbows and upper arms at your sides, bring weights up toward the ceiling. Slowly bring arms back to starting position, keeping your leg lifted.

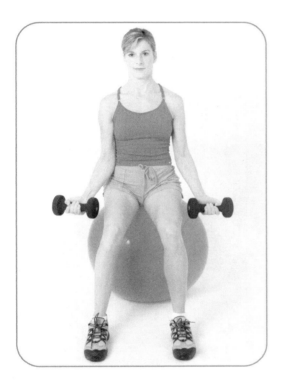
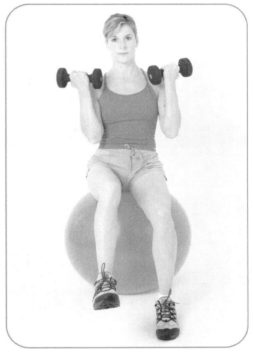

HAMMER CURL WITH BAND

Stand straight, holding the resistance band with palms facing inward. Step on the resistance band so that there is an even amount of tubing on each side. Begin with your arms straight down and slightly in front of your body. Keeping your elbows and upper arms at your sides, bring arms up toward the ceiling. Slowly bring arms back to starting position.

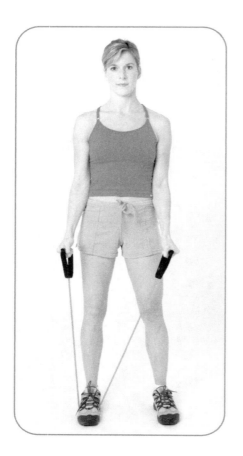 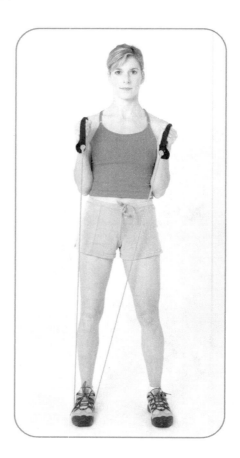

TRICEPS PUSH-DOWN

Sit upright on the ball with your legs in front of you. Hold the weight directly over your head with both hands, palms facing toward the ceiling, thumbs interlaced. Begin with the weight directly over your head, elbows slightly bent. Lift one leg off the floor a few inches. Lower weight behind you until your elbows are at a 90-degree angle. Slowly bring weight back to starting position, keeping your leg lifted.

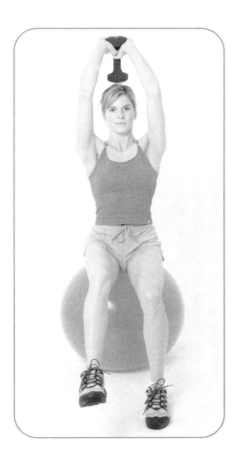 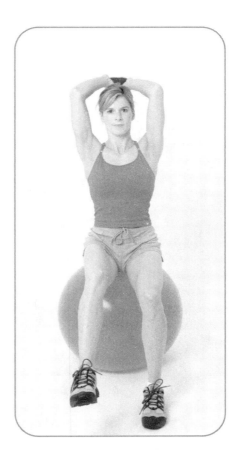

TRICEPS DIP OFF BALL

Start by sitting on the ball, feet in front of you. Lift yourself off the ball with the palms of your hands balanced on the ball. Dip straight down to the floor, bending at the elbows. Lift yourself back up to starting position.

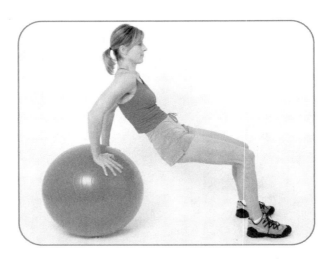

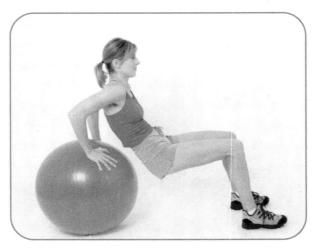

KICKBACK ON BALL

Lie with your torso on the ball, legs extended out behind you. Keep your back straight throughout the exercise. Begin with your arms at your sides, elbows bent at a 90-degree angle so that your hands are next to the ball. Straighten out arms at your sides, keeping your elbows and upper arms still. Slowly bring your arms back to starting position.

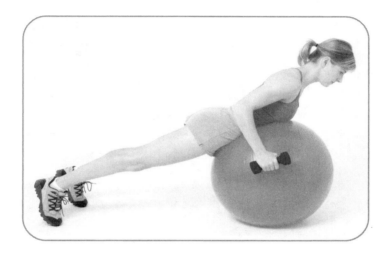

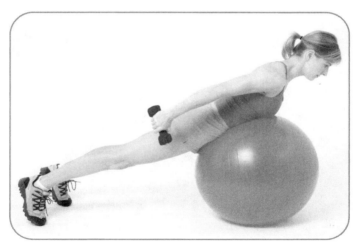

EXERCISE BALL CRUNCH THREE

Lie with your back on the ball and your feet securely on the wall. Place your hands behind your ears. Begin with your body extended over the ball. Lift your shoulder blades off the ball and up toward the ceiling. Slowly bring yourself back to the starting position.

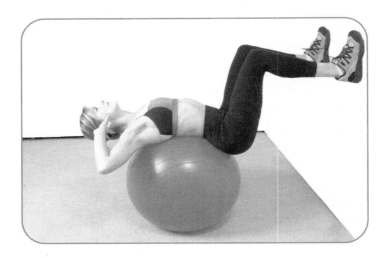

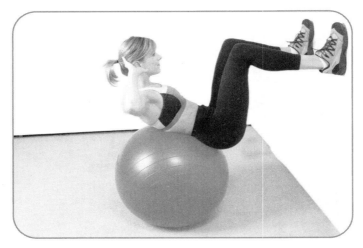

BIKE ON BALL

Lie on the floor with the heels of your feet on the ball. Place your hands behind your ears. Lift your shoulder blades off the floor. Bring one knee toward your chest and rotate your upper body, bringing your opposite elbow to your knee. Repeat on the other side.

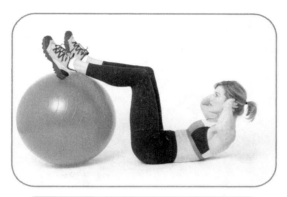

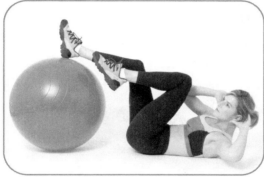

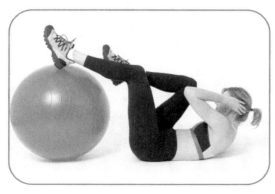

OBLIQUE ON BALL

Lie on your side with your torso on the ball, feet securely against the wall. Place one hand on your head and your other hand on your hip. Lift your torso off the ball, toward the wall. Slowly bring your torso back down to starting position. Repeat on the other side.

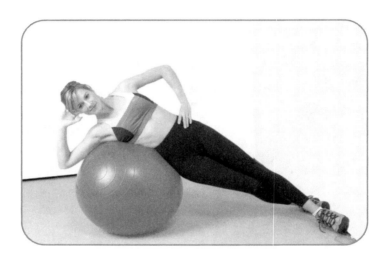

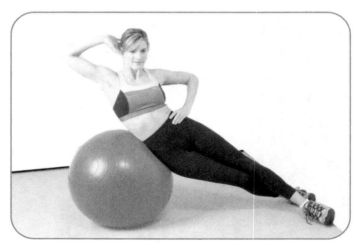

ROLLING JACKKNIFE

Begin with your feet and shins on the ball and your arms shoulder width apart on the floor. Straighten out your back, making a plank with your body. Using your abdominal muscles, pull the ball toward you, bringing your knees to your chest. Slowly bring the ball back to starting position.

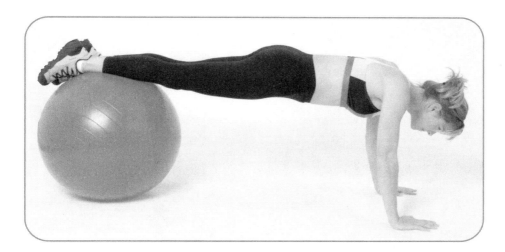

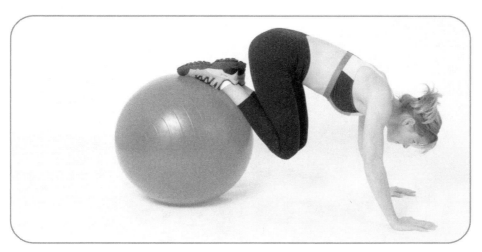

KAYAKER WITH LEGS

Balancing on your butt, create a V with your body by lifting your feet off the floor and leaning back with your upper body. Place a weight in your hands, palms facing inward. Touch the weight side to side on the floor by rotating your torso. At the same time, extend the leg on the opposite side of your body.

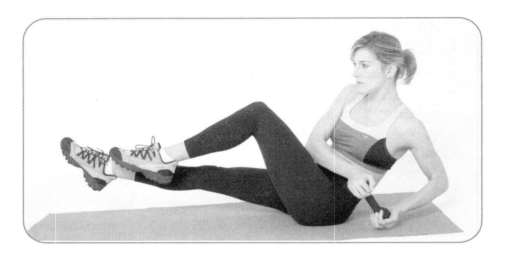

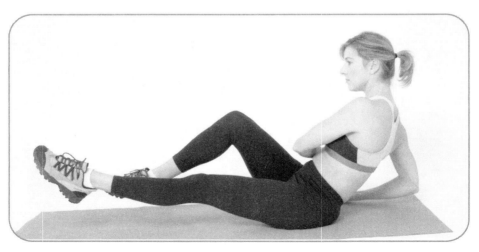

ROTATING PLANK

Start in a straight push-up position, legs close together and hands shoulder width apart on the floor. Maintain a straight torso and hips throughout the exercise. Rotate to one side, keeping one arm underneath you as the other arm extends toward the ceiling. Hold for a few seconds. Slowly bring your body back to starting position, then repeat on the other side.

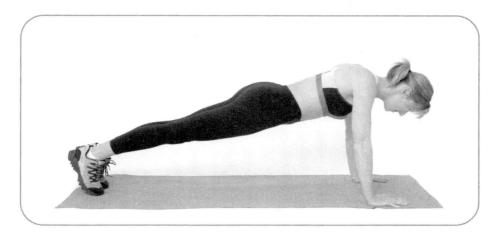

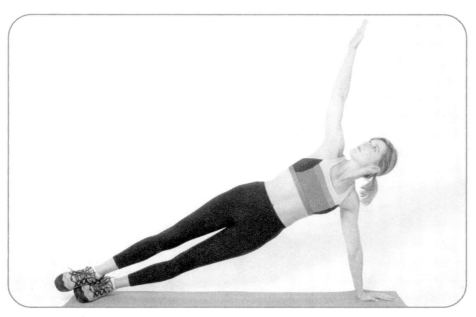

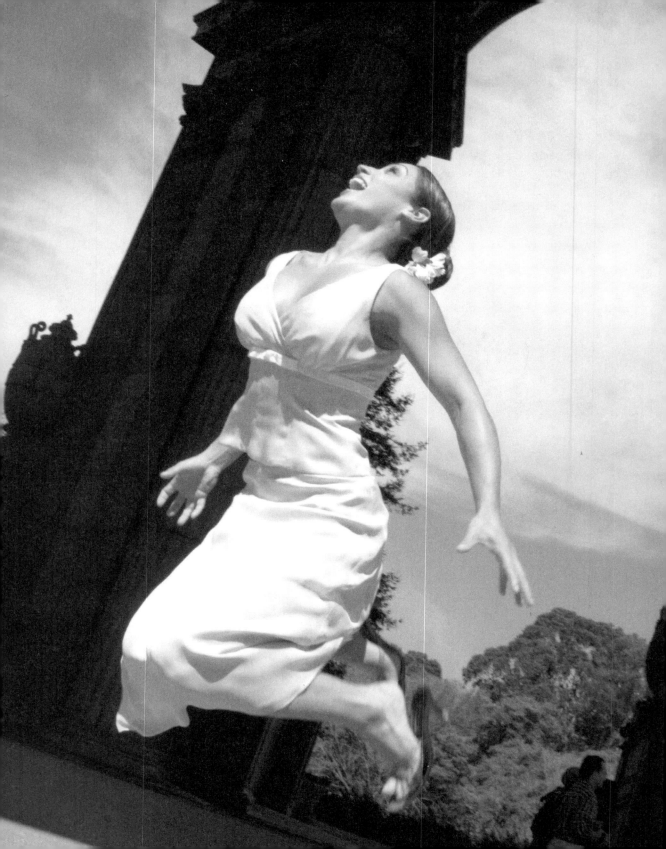

THE BRIDE'S ONE-HOUR FULL-BODY WORKOUT

WORKOUT FOR THE WEEK OF YOUR WEDDING

Only one week to go before your big day! Out-of-town family and friends are arriving, the caterer is calling for a final head count, and you've got to pack for your honeymoon. You've also had your final dress fitting and you want to ensure that it looks as fantastic on you as it does right now. I can tell you from experience that this isn't the time to skip your workouts. Exercise relieves stress, and right now you need all the stress relief you can get. With that said, I know firsthand that family and vendor commitments make it hard to get away to the gym.

Real Brides: Tips from the Trenches

Accentuate your assets. You've worked hard, dripped with sweat on the elliptical machine, lifted many pounds of weights, and sculpted a lean upper body. Emphasize your physique by adding a small two-pound weight inside your bridal bouquet. Your muscles will be flexed as you walk down the aisle, highlighting the definition in your arms.

The Bride's One-Hour Full-Body Workout combines all the essential elements of fitness to give you the best full-body workout in just one hour. This routine was developed by one of our best drill sergeants, Amy Holley, and every bride can do it. This workout was designed specifically for that special week and day of your wedding. You can do this workout anywhere: bedroom, basement, parents' house, or hotel room. As with all of our workouts, I have put a log in the appendix so that you can have all the exercises at your fingertips and can track your progress through the week. For the week of your wedding, do this workout *every morning*. When you wake up the morning of your wedding, hopefully after a good night's sleep, do this workout first thing before you start getting ready and before the makeup and hair stylists arrive. Perhaps your maid of honor will work out with you. Trust me, you will be so thankful that you did it. Your nerves will be at rest and your mind will be filled with confidence.

The Bride's One-Hour Full-Body Workout combines aerobic and strength training to give you everything you need to tone up and burn fat. You will perform exercises for every major muscle group for five minutes at a time. Strength training with a band for five minutes, instead of doing thirty repetitions, creates a workout that is as much aerobic as it is strength training. In between every major-muscle-group exercise, you will do one minute of high-intensity aerobic intervals such as running in place or jumping jacks. High-intensity intervals keep the heart rate up and your body in the fat-burning zone.

During the five minutes of biceps curls, lunges, and other exercises, you should vary the tempo every minute or so. Varying tempos, such as one second down, one second up, and then three seconds up and one second down, will work your muscles slightly differently every time. Think of it as slowing down and speeding up every time you perform one repetition. Trust me, you will feel the burn!

Keep your resistance band next to your bed so that you won't forget it. You've come so far and you aren't about to let it all go this close to your wedding day. You have finally arrived and it's time to show off your new shapely, toned body! Look in the mirror—you look amazing!

WARM-UP	50 jumping jacks	Stay light on your feet and easy on your joints. Make sure to move your arms
WARM-UP	20 squats	Legs wide, reach hips back, keep knees over ankles
WARM-UP	20 lunges, each leg	Keep knees over ankles, reach hips straight down to the floor, back straight
1 MINUTE	Stretch	All major muscle groups: quads, hamstrings, chest, back (upper and lower), shoulders, biceps, triceps, calves
5 MINUTES	Squats	Vary tempo: 1/1, 3/1, 1/3, 4/4
1 MINUTE	Jump rope	If no rope, still move arms and legs to keep up the intensity
5 MINUTES	Chest	Push-ups Flies with band Vary tempo: 1/1, 3/1, 1/3, 4/4
1 MINUTE	Run in place	Run
5 MINUTES	Triceps	Kickbacks with band Vary tempo: 1/1, 3/1, 1/3, 4/4
1 MINUTE	Jump rope	If no rope, still move arms and legs to keep up the intensity
5 MINUTES	Lunges	Backward lunges Vary tempo: 1/1, 3/1, 1/3, 4/4
1 MINUTE	Jumping jacks	Vary tempo: 1/1, 3/1, 1/3, 4/4
5 MINUTES	Back	Rows with band. Use a railing or a pipe for band Vary tempo: 1/1, 3/1, 1/3, 4/4
1 MINUTE	Squat 180	Squat and jump, squat and jump
5 MINUTES	Biceps	Biceps curl with band under one foot Vary tempo: 1/1, 3/1, 1/3, 4/4 Vary range of motion: half up, half down, hold in middle, pulse
1 MINUTE	Jumping jacks	Stand straight, keeping your knees slightly bent throughout exercise.
5 MINUTES	Shoulders	Overhead press Vary tempo: 1/1, 3/1, 1/3, 4/4
10 MINUTES	Abs/lower back	Crunches, reverse curls, bicycles, planks, back extension (swimmer)
5 MINUTES	Stretch/cool down	All major muscle groups: quads, hamstrings, chest, back (upper and lower), shoulders, biceps, triceps, calves

JUMPING JACKS

Stand, legs together with arms directly at your sides. Jump out, bringing your arms over your head, and immediately jump back to starting position.

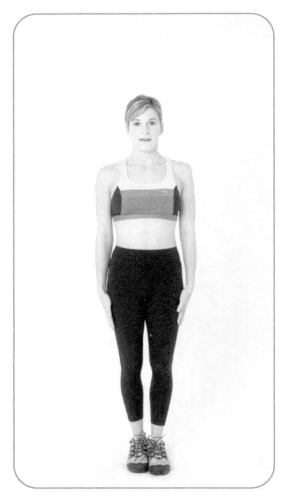
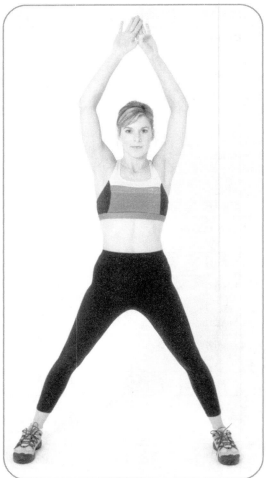

SQUATS

Stand with legs slightly wider than hip width apart, arms in front of you at chest level for balance. Squat down, sticking your butt out as if you are trying to sit down. Do not let your knees go beyond your ankles. Slowly bring yourself back to starting position.

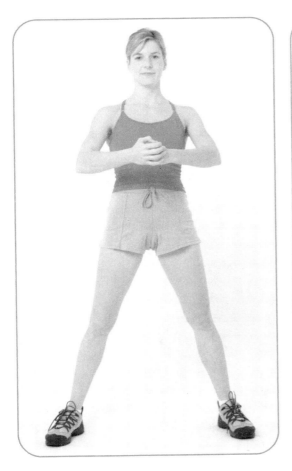
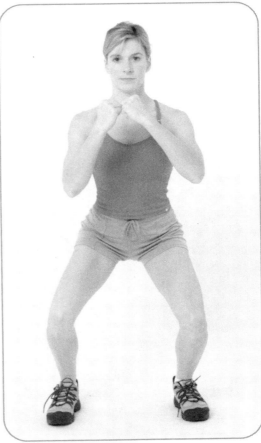

LUNGES

Stand straight, arms at your sides, feet facing forward. Bring one leg far enough in front of you to perform a lunge. Dip straight down to the floor, bending both knees and keeping the back straight. Do not let your knee go beyond your ankle. With control, bring your body back to starting position. Repeat on the other side.

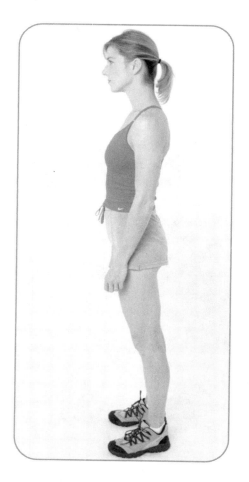 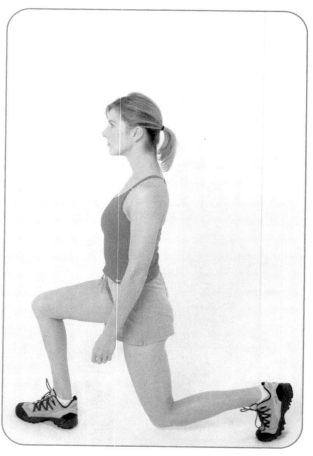

STRETCH: Stretch all major muscle groups before starting exercises.

SQUATS

Stand with legs slightly wider than hip width apart, arms in front of you at chest level for balance. Squat down, sticking your butt out as if you are sitting in a chair. Do not let your knees go beyond your ankles. With control, bring yourself back to starting position. Vary tempo: 1 second down, 1 second up; 3 seconds down, 1 second up; 1 second down, 3 seconds up; 4 seconds down, 4 seconds up.

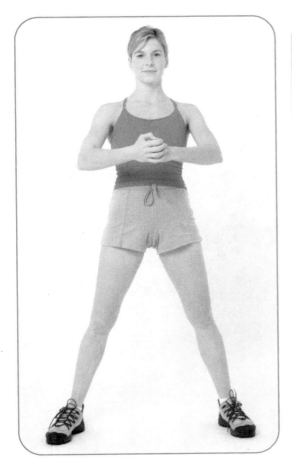
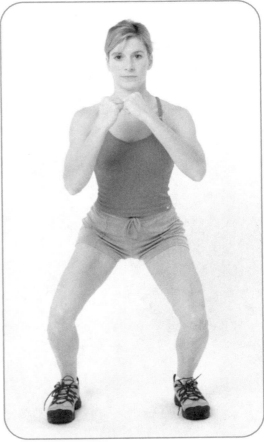

JUMP ROPE

Stand straight, keeping your knees slightly bent throughout the exercise. Jump rope.

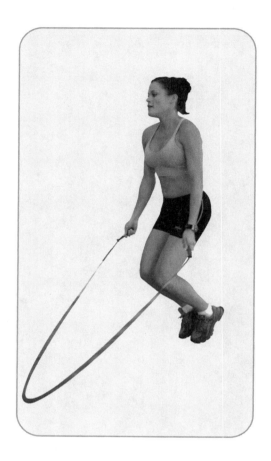

KNEE PUSH-UP

Place knees close together on the floor. Hands should be slightly farther than shoulder width apart. Keep your feet on the floor behind you, back straight. Begin upright with arms straight. Lower yourself so that your nose can almost touch the floor. Slowly bring yourself back to starting position.

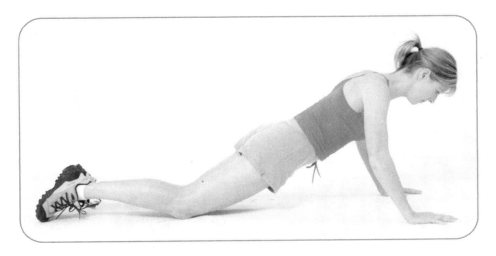

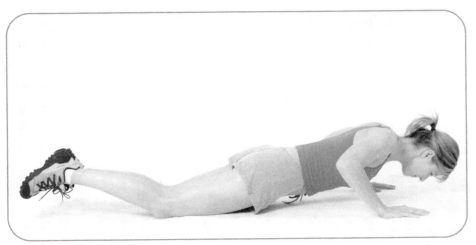

RESISTANCE BAND CHEST FLIES

Wrap the band around your back at chest level, holding below the handles, palms facing downward. Keep arms at chest level throughout the exercise. Bring your arms forward as if you have a big ball in front of your chest. Slowly, bring your arms back to starting position. Vary tempo: 1 second out, 1 second back; 3 seconds out, 1 second back; 1 second out, 3 seconds back; 4 seconds out, 4 seconds back.

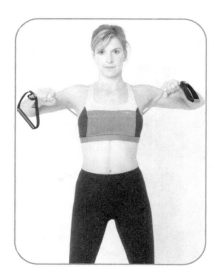 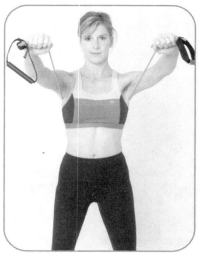

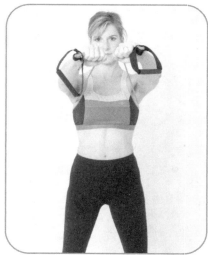

RUN IN PLACE

Run in place. Switch between knees up in front of you and kicking your butt with your feet.

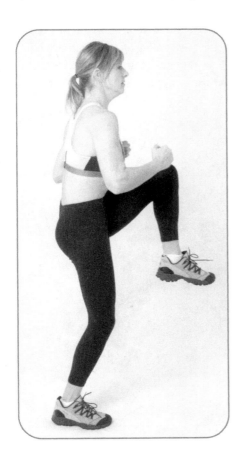 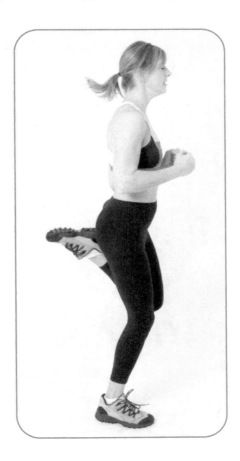

KICKBACKS WITH BAND

Stand straight with feet together, knees bent. Bend over so that your back is straight by sticking out your chest and butt. Place one end of the band underneath your feet, holding the band with your hand, palm facing your body. Begin with your arm directly at your side, elbow bent at a 90-degree angle. Straighten out your arm at your side, keeping your elbow and upper arm still. Slowly bring your arm back to starting position. Vary tempo: 1 second out, 1 second back; 3 seconds out, 1 second back; 1 second out, 3 seconds back; 4 seconds out, 4 seconds back. Repeat on the other side.

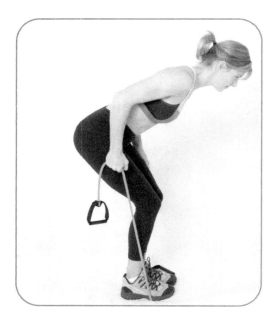 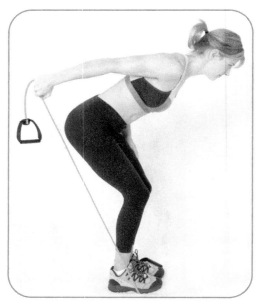

JUMP ROPE

Stand straight, keeping your knees slightly bent throughout the exercise. Jump rope.

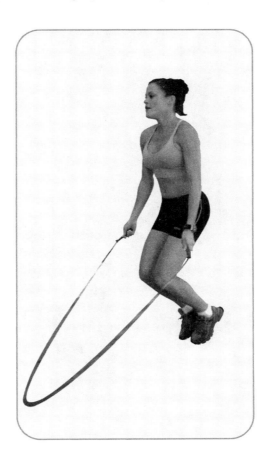

BACKWARD LUNGES

Stand straight with both feet facing forward, arms at your sides. Keeping your upper body straight, place your leg straight behind you, far enough back to perform a lunge. Dip straight down, bending both knees. Do not let your front knee go beyond your ankle. Lift straight up, bringing your leg back to starting position. Vary tempo: 1 second down, 1 second up; 3 seconds down, 1 second up; 1 second down, 3 seconds up; 4 seconds down, 4 seconds up. Repeat on the other side.

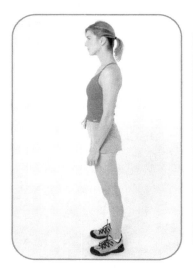 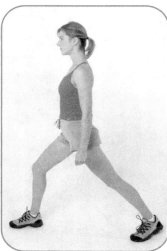 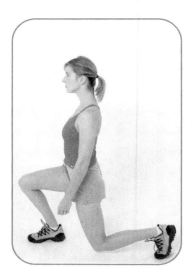

JUMPING JACKS

Stand, legs together with arms directly at your sides. Jump out, bringing your arms over your head, and immediately jump back to starting position.

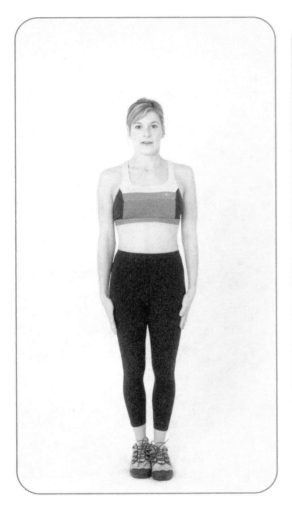
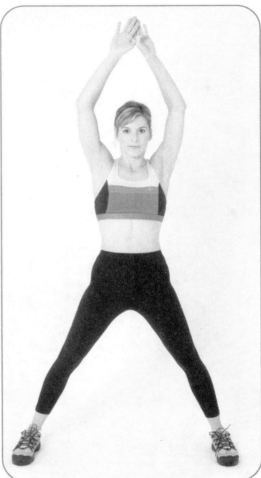

ROWS

Tie the center of the resistance band to a doorknob, or lace it around a pole or stairwell railing. Stand straight with one leg slightly behind you for balance. Begin by holding on to the band at chest level, arms straight. Bring your arms back, squeezing your shoulder blades together. With control, bring your arms back to starting position. Vary tempo: 1 second back, 1 second forward; 3 seconds back, 1 second forward; 1 second back, 3 seconds forward; 4 seconds back, 4 seconds forward.

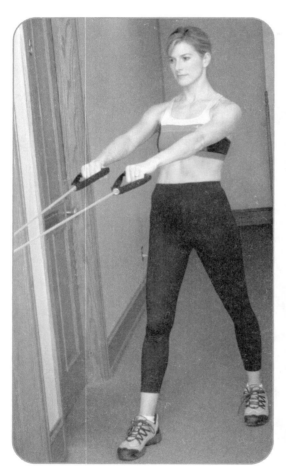 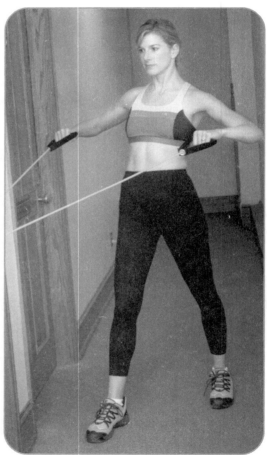

SQUAT 180

Stand straight with legs wider than hip width apart. Keep your arms close to your sides for balance. Jump up and to the side, gently landing on your feet, legs still wider than hip width apart. Squat down, sticking your butt out as if you are trying to sit down. Bring your body back up and jump and rotate to the other side. Repeat the squat. Continue to jump side to side, squatting on each side.

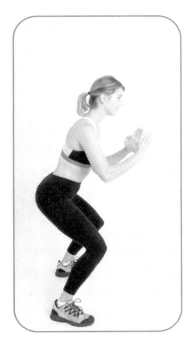 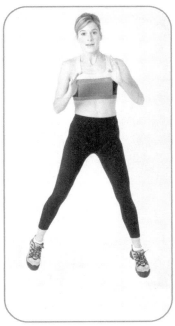 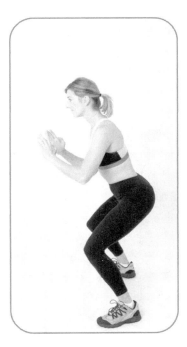

BICEPS CURL WITH BAND

Stand straight, legs hip width apart. Place the center of the band under your foot so that there is an even amount of tubing on each side. Hold the band with palms facing forward. Begin with arms straight down at your sides. Keep your elbows and upper arms glued to the sides of your body throughout the exercise. Bring the band up to your shoulders by bending your elbows. With control, bring the band back to starting position. Vary tempo: 1 second up, 1 second down; 3 seconds up, 1 second down; 1 second up, 3 seconds down; 4 seconds up, 4 seconds down. Vary range of motion: half up, half down, hold in middle, pulse.

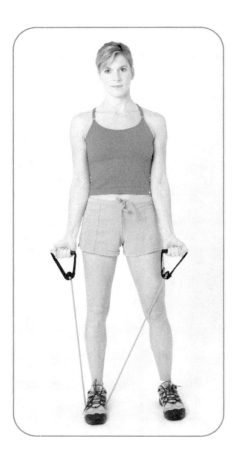 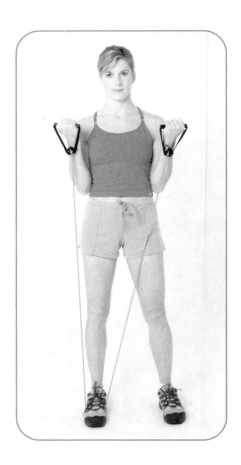

JUMPING JACKS

Stand, legs together with arms directly at your sides. Jump out, bringing your arms over your head, and immediately jump back to starting position.

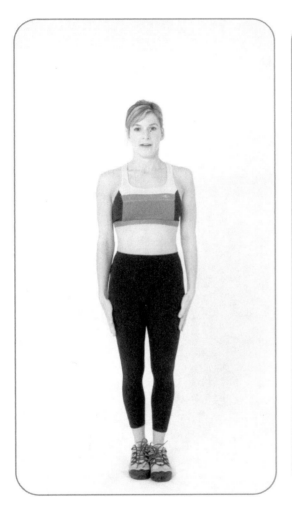
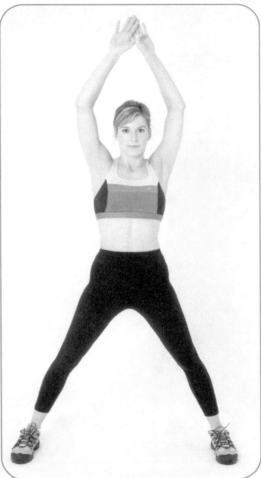

OVERHEAD PRESS

Hold the handles of the band, palms facing inward. Step on the band so that you have an even amount of tubing on both sides. Begin with your arms at shoulder level, elbows at a 90-degree angle. Lift arms upward and inward toward the ceiling. Slowly bring arms back down to starting position. Make sure not to lower your arms past your shoulder level. Vary tempo: 1 second up, 1 second down; 3 seconds up, 1 second down; 1 second up, 3 seconds down; 4 seconds up, 4 seconds down.

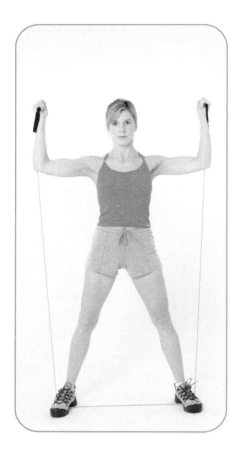 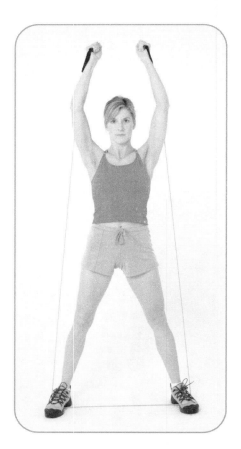

ABS

Vary abs: crunches, reverse curls, bicycles, planks, back extension (swimmer). Do abs for 10 minutes.

STRETCH

Stretch all major muscle groups: quads, hamstrings, chest, back (upper and lower), shoulders, biceps, triceps, calves.

CONGRATULATIONS AND BEST WISHES! Remember, you have worked hard to get where you are today. You have officially been promoted from recruit to active duty. I look forward to seeing you again in Reserves.

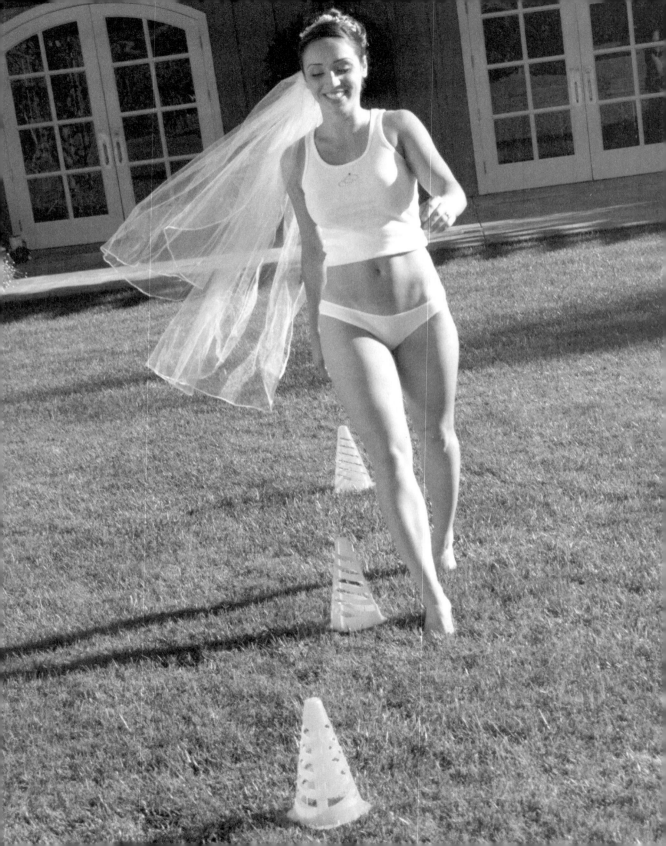

BOOTCAMP360 FUEL

GEARING UP: NUTRITION

The adage "You are what you eat" is absolutely true. It is especially true for brides who want radiant skin, shiny hair, and a toned body for their big day in front of their closest friends and family (and some guests that you have never met before!). Don't forget about all the energy you need—planning your wedding, dealing with overly involved family, and balancing time and money.

Eating healthy is one of the toughest challenges for most people. Feelings of frustration and stress can easily lead to overeating and emotional bingeing. This is the time to break the unhealthy habits and get your nutrition under control.

From here on out you will view food not only as an enjoyable social experience or an emotional crutch, but as fuel for an active body. When someone bakes a batch of cookies, how many can you eat? It's almost endless, isn't it? You can easily eat a half dozen and probably more. But you can't eat five or six apples. You would be way too full to eat that many because apples, unlike cookies, are low in calories but high in nutritional value. The same applies to the bread that they serve you in restaurants. How many pieces can you eat before your appetizer even arrives? Most of us can eat an entire loaf of bread and still be hungry, but if you ate that much fish or chicken, you would be completely full. You get the point. You need to make smart choices.

BOOTCAMP360 SUCCESS STORY

RECRUIT KRISTA

POUNDS LOST: 22
INCHES LOST: 13
BODY FAT % LOST: 7

SOMETHING OLD

SOMETHING NEW

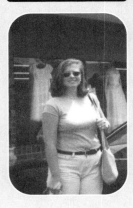 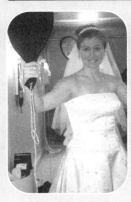 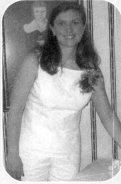

When I got engaged, I felt beautiful and awful at the same time. I had no energy and constantly felt discouraged about the way I looked. I knew I could look a lot better, and at that point I became bound and determined to lose weight and tone up my body.

I knew I wanted to lose weight but felt completely unmotivated. That's why I joined Bootcamp360 for Brides; I needed someone to give me a quick kick in the butt! For once I wanted to be treated like an athlete, not a helpless girl. I finally found something that didn't let me make excuses, that made me look at myself and my actions honestly. I could no longer hide behind my lazy ways. It was the "no excuses" attitude that drove my success. I truly felt that I was in training and not on a diet-and-exercise program. Because of this, I took it seriously and whipped my butt back into shape. I no longer let myself get away with my old habits, and view exercise and eating healthy as a lifelong change . . . after all, I am an athlete now!

I started the program the minute my fiancé proposed, so I have yet to walk down the aisle. However, as I inch closer to my wedding date, I no longer have to stress out about being overweight or self-conscious. I took care of that months ago. Now I can focus on being creative and planning the perfect day.

Each bride is unique, and while some have the time to make their lunch the night before, others eat out daily. The key is to find the healthiest, most convenient choices that work for you.

Incorporating the "I do's" of nutrition into your eating habits will keep your energy strong, your body balanced, and your skin and hair glowing.

"I Do's" of Nutrition

I Do #1: Drink H_2O
I Do #2: Control Your Portions
I Do #3: Eat Your Greens and Your Fruits
I Do #4: Dinner Difference
I Do #5: Fats Are Good
I Do #6: Cut Out Caffeine
I Do #7: Alcohol in Moderation
I Do #8: Fuel Up for Exercise

I DO #1: DRINK H_2O   Drink up if you want to avoid pesky pimples or blotches on your wedding day.

Water makes up approximately 70 percent of the body and is the most important nutrient. Your body can only absorb about eight ounces at one time, so you need to drink throughout the day. You should drink at least ten to twelve 8-ounce glasses daily. Get into the habit of having your water bottle at your side at all times. It is especially important to stay hydrated when you exercise. Remember, a hydrated body is lean and toned, while a dehydrated body is bloated. Water is extremely important in flushing toxins from the body, and the key to clear, healthy skin.

I DO #2: CONTROL YOUR PORTIONS   Did you grow up having to eat everything on your plate? Some habits are born out of our childhood and carry on to our new families. A drill sergeant made a good point that caused many recruits to realize that not finishing every bite on your plate is actually a good thing. She pointed out that if you consume calories that you don't need, your body doesn't use them and they go to waste. The excess food can either go to waste on your hips or thighs, or in the garbage. You don't have to throw food away: put leftovers in the fridge for another meal when you need the fuel again. Don't let excess food go to waste on your body!

Your hand is the best indicator of portions. The palm of your hand is a portion of pasta, grains, or rice. The flat part of the palm of your hand, or a deck of cards, is a portion of fish or meat. One portion of cheese is only equal to the upper part of your thumb. Keep these portions in mind when you are eating your next meal. I bet you will find, as many recruits do, that your portions are a lot larger than you ever thought. That equates to a lot more calories than you ever thought were going into your body.

Real Brides: Tips from the Trenches

Drink a glass of water before every meal. You will start your meal somewhat full. Between every bite, put your fork down and take another sip of water. It will keep you hydrated and full while decreasing your chances of unsightly blemishes. —*Recruit Jessica*

In reality, food is a fuel source for the body, not just the center of social occasions. You can't drive your car on empty. Your body works in much the same way, and the goal here is to give your body the right fuel consistently throughout the day.

The average adult woman needs approximately 1,200 to 1,600 nutritious calories daily. For your exact caloric needs, speak to your doctor. If your goal is to eat 1,600 calories daily, divide that by the number of meals you eat in a day.

You should be eating four to five small balanced meals every day. Pick foods that are packed with nutrients: fruits, vegetables, fish, chicken, grains, and legumes. You will fill up quickly and your body will thank you with higher levels of energy.

Real Brides: Tips from the Trenches

Eat a healthy snack before attending your bridal shower and you won't be tempted to try every sweet there. Since everyone is there to see you, it's nice to spend the time chatting with your guests, rather than filling your face. Let the guests enjoy the food and spend much-desired time with you, the bride-to-be. —*Recruit Krista*

Each meal should contain healthy carbohydrate, protein, and fat. The body looks to carbohydrates first as its main fuel source. That's why many people who are on low-carb diets feel lethargic and lack energy. The body stores only a limited amount of glycogen, and it is the only source of fuel for the nervous system and brain, along with providing energy for such tasks as strength training. Vegetables, whole grains, and fruit are excellent sources of carbohydrates and provide valuable energy and nutrients. Healthy fats such as olive oil have proven to be both satisfying and good for the heart. Protein is essential for rebuilding muscle and is the last source of energy for the body behind carbohydrates and fats. Protein should be an important part of every meal, especially when exercising regularly.

Real Brides: Tips from the Trenches

Serve dinner on an appetizer plate. My fiancé cooks most nights, which means lots of food piled high onto the plate. I went to the local department store and bought a set of appetizer plates. For the first few months I hid our normal plates, forcing my fiancé to serve dinner on the smaller plates. He still piled it high, but it was half the food he normally serves. We both lost weight thanks to my little trick. —*Recruit Anna*

Have you ever left a restaurant feeling so full that you are convinced you are going to pop? Me too. The bottom line is that your portions are more than likely too large—your body doesn't need an entire plate of pasta or rice.

Eating out doesn't mean eating everything. Simply take the temptation away. Out of sight is truly out of mind. When you sit down, ask the waiter to refrain from bringing you the tempting bread basket, or ask him or her to put half of your entrée in a to-go box before it even reaches the table. Most of us won't finish everything on our plate. Take it home, store it, then eat it for lunch the next day. Think of it as getting two meals for the price of one.

Real Brides: Tips from the Trenches

When dining out, order two appetizers instead of one main course. That way, you get a variety of tastes, but smaller portions. Get one appetizer that is heavier on the good carbs and one that is heavier on the protein. You will end up with a balanced and healthy meal. —*Recruit Michelle*

When ordering out, we have much less control over the preparation of our meals. As a consequence, we unknowingly eat more saturated fats and salt. This leaves us at risk for not getting necessary nutrients while increasing our caloric intake dramatically. The next time you order, make it a point to ask the waiter to hold the butter and salt, even if it isn't specifically listed on the menu. You will taste and feel the difference immediately.

I DO #3: EAT YOUR GREENS AND YOUR FRUITS

Make sure your plate is always packed with vegetables. You can't always count calories or control portions, but you can visually make the right decisions. Vegetables such as kale, broccoli, and collards are packed full of nutrients, including calcium, which is an important mineral for women. Always try to fill at least half of your plate with veggies. Consider veggies your main dish and chicken your side dish, not the other way around. You will fill up a lot faster and your energy levels will soar all day. Fibrous vegetables such as leafy greens also keep your body regular, a positive side benefit.

Eat your roughage if you want to bypass the bloated blahs on your wedding day. If you've ever started the day feeling slim and comfortable in your clothes, but feel that you need to unbutton your pants at some point throughout the day, you are probably feeling bloated. Drinking water will help, and so will eating fibrous foods, such as vegetables and fruits.

Fruit is truly Mother Nature's gift, acting as a natural detoxifier for the body. Eat at least two portions a day. A small orange, apple, or pear equals one portion. Ten cherries or strawberries are also one portion. Eat one portion of fruit as a morning snack and one as an after-lunch snack. Add some canned tuna (packed in water) or edamame (nuts are really a fat source) for your protein. The combination makes a perfect small meal.

I DO #4: DINNER DIFFERENCE

Dinner should always be a serving of protein over fibrous veggies, such as salmon over spinach or chicken on a bed of broccoli and squash. You'll see a dramatic difference in your weight-loss efforts, and you'll also sleep better when you body isn't trying to digest processed carbohydrates.

A rule to live by is no simple carbohydrates after 3 p.m. What does this mean? No bread, rice, pasta, or fruit after 3 p.m. You should eat your simple carbohydrates earlier in the day when you can use the energy. Eating simple carbohydrates late at night leaves your body with lots of fuel and nowhere to use it. Unlike cars, which use it the next day, we store the unused fuel as fat in our bodies and then need to refuel again.

Your body does a lot of its repair work at night while you are sleeping, so feed it protein at dinner. Protein is essential for rebuilding muscle and tissue. As you put more pressure on your body, you want to make sure that you are getting enough protein. Don't worry about trying to weigh your protein; instead, fill one-third of your plate with protein every meal.

PROTEIN-RICH FOODS	SERVING SIZE
Low-fat cottage cheese	½ cup
Edamame	⅔ cup, shelled
Salmon	Palm of your hand
Skinless chicken	Palm of your hand
Tofu	1-inch cube

I DO #5: FATS ARE GOOD   Eating (healthy) fats doesn't have to mean feeling fat in your wedding dress. Whoever told you that all fats are bad was just plain wrong. Fats are the building blocks of the body and are important for many major functions. However, this doesn't mean that you should deep-fry all of your dinners and eat cheesecake for breakfast. Not all fats are created equal; some are really good for you, while others are not.

Monounsaturated fats such as olive oil, avocado, sesame oil, nuts, and the fat found in fish are incredibly healthy and should be an important part of your diet. Add a little of these fats to each meal for flavor and fuel. Fat also triggers satiety in your body. Adding a little olive oil to your steamed vegetables will not only make them taste better but will also trigger your brain into thinking it's full a lot faster, and you won't finish your plate of veggies wanting to scour the fridge for goodies.

I DO #6: CUT OUT CAFFEINE   Plain and simple, caffeine is a weight-loss inhibitor. Not only does it impede digestion, but it is also hard on the liver, your body's detoxifying organ. It can also create a not-so-attractive puffiness in your face. Cut out caffeine as much as you can. If you drink coffee every morning, try to brew or order it with half decaf.

Of course, drink more water than soda. Sometimes your body thinks it's tired and needs caffeine when it is really dehydrated and needs water. Before you reach for a soda or coffee after lunch, try some water first. You may find that you don't need the caffeine after all. The combination of stress and caffeine can turn you from a lovely bride into a crazed, moody bride. Don't let that happen to you.

I DO #7: ALCOHOL IN MODERATION Alcohol has a lot of calories. Having a few glasses of wine or beer with dinner can add up to thousands of extra calories. It can also lower your inhibitions, making that piece of chocolate mousse cake look appetizing. Drink alcohol in moderation and on special occasions only, and when you do drink, try alternating between a glass of wine and a glass of water. Your once-in-a-lifetime bachelorette party definitely counts as a special occasion worthy of a drink or two with your girlfriends!

Real Brides: Tips from the Trenches

Walk it off! It's your big day and the butterflies in your stomach are all aflutter. Calm your nerves by taking a quick, brisk walk in the early morning. You will return calm, collected, and ready for the chaos. —*Recruit Denise*

I DO #8: FUEL UP FOR EXERCISE Eating before exercise is essential to getting the most out of your workout. Never go into exercise hungry. You need to make sure that you haven't depleted your body before you begin. Make sure to have a small meal (two hundred to three hundred calories) a couple of hours before you exercise. If you are exercising after work, but before dinner, eat a healthy snack containing protein and carbohydrates. Nutritional bars are an easy option that you can keep in your desk or purse. If working out first thing in the morning, have a banana and some natural peanut butter. You need to eat enough to take away the grumbling in your stomach, but not so much that you are too full to exercise.

BOOTCAMP360 MESS HALL RECIPES
16 Ingredients, 42 Scrumptious Recipes

The key to success, especially with nutrition, is to stave off the boredom. The following delicious recipes will please the palate and keep you trim without breaking the bank. The numbers were derived from average calories for foods. Calories for various brands may vary. Please read the labels of foods purchased. And remember—these recipes can be paired up to make a fabulous meal. For example, start with the gazpacho as an appetizer and have the lemon chicken, or have a serving of the omelet with a side of salsa.

STOCKED PANTRY   There are a few ingredients you should always keep in the pantry: olive oil for cooking and for dressings, cornstarch for thickening, low-sodium chicken broth for a soup base, salt and pepper for seasoning, and your favorite dried herbs and spices (thyme, oregano, basil, etc.). As long as you have these ingredients handy, you can always make a meal.

GROCERY LIST   The Bootcamp360 grocery list is designed for ease, convenience, and taste. These ingredients provide the good carbohydrates, proteins, and healthy fats you need to lose weight and tone up. The beauty about all these recipes is that you can substitute many of your favorite ingredients while maintaining the delicious flavor and healthy balance. The table below includes your main grocery list as well as a potential substitution list. These recipes also include optional ingredients (*) that may enhance the flavor but are not necessary. Enjoy!

GROCERY LIST	POSSIBLE SUBSTITUTION LIST	GROCERY LIST (CONT.)	POSSIBLE SUBSTITUTION LIST
Quinoa (grain)	Couscous/barley/brown rice	Eggs	Egg whites
Chicken	Turkey/lamb/buffalo meat	Mushrooms	Any type of mushroom
Tuna (canned or fresh)	Any white fish/salmon	Onions	Any type of onion
Red peppers	Squash/zucchini/yellow & green peppers	Spinach	Kale/any type of lettuce
Tomato		Garbanzo beans	White beans
Avocado		Feta cheese	Goat cheese Parmesan cheese
Lemon	Lime	Whole-wheat pita	Whole-wheat bread
Orange	Mango/papaya/other citrus fruits	Cucumber	

BREAKFAST

Scrambled Eggs with Spinach, Red Peppers, and Mushrooms

---

5 TEASPOONS OLIVE OIL
12 MUSHROOMS, STEMMED AND SLICED
¾ CUP CHOPPED ONIONS
1 CUP COARSELY CHOPPED RED BELL PEPPERS
1½ CUPS CHOPPED FRESH SPINACH
1 TEASPOON CHOPPED FRESH THYME*
6 EGG WHITES

Makes 2 servings servings
237 calories per serving

Heat 1 teaspoon of the olive oil in a large non-stick skillet over medium-high heat. Add the mushrooms and cook until soft, stirring frequently. Set the mushrooms aside, covered by paper towels.

Meanwhile, heat 3 teaspoons of the oil in a large nonstick skillet over medium heat. Add the onions and red bell peppers, and sauté until soft and brown, 3 to 4 minutes. Add the spinach; toss until wilted, about 3 minutes. Stir in the optional thyme. Set the onions and peppers and spinach aside, covered by paper towels.

Whisk the egg whites in a medium bowl. Sprinkle with salt and pepper. Heat the remaining 1 teaspoon of oil in a medium nonstick skillet over medium heat. Pour the eggs into the skillet; stir until softly set, about 2 minutes. Add the mushrooms, onions and peppers, and spinach. Stir gently until cooked. Serve immediately.

Spinach, Red Pepper, and Egg Muffins

9 EGG WHITES
1 TEASPOON GROUND BLACK PEPPER
¼ CUP FINELY CHOPPED RED BELL PEPPER
½ CUP CHOPPED FRESH SPINACH, COOKED
2 TABLESPOONS CRUMBLED FETA CHEESE*

Makes 4 egg muffins
66 calories per serving

Preheat the oven to 325°F. Coat a muffin pan with a nonstick, nonfat spray or use muffin cups.

Whisk the egg whites and black pepper together in a medium bowl. Add the red peppers and spinach (make sure the spinach is cooked until wilted prior to adding it to the mixture). Mix thoroughly. Gently add in the feta cheese, if desired. Fill the muffin cups halfway. Bake until the egg is completely cooked, 20 to 25 minutes. Serve warm or store in the fridge for a later time.

Spicy Scrambled Eggs

⅔ CUP SALSA (RECIPE PAGE 216 OR STORE-BOUGHT)
½ CUP CANNED GARBANZO BEANS (CHICKPEAS), RINSED AND DRAINED
2 TABLESPOONS DRIED CILANTRO*
GROUND BLACK PEPPER
2 WHOLE-WHEAT PITAS
8 EGG WHITES
MILK*

Makes 4 servings
278 calories per serving

Stir together the salsa, beans, and cilantro in a medium bowl.

Add black pepper to taste.

Cut the pitas into halves. Whip the egg whites in a medium bowl. Season with pepper to taste. If you like your eggs a little more fluffy, add 1 tablespoon milk. Pour the eggs into a medium nonstick skillet over medium heat. Cover and let cook until lightly set. Gently lift the sides with a spatula and let the uncooked eggs slide to the bottom of the pan. Cover and let cook for another 5 minutes, or until the eggs are cooked through. Cut into four pieces. Place one piece in each pita half and cover with the salsa mixture.

Baked Eggs with Spinach

½ **ONION, FINELY CHOPPED**
1 **TABLESPOON OLIVE OIL**
3 **CUPS COARSELY CHOPPED FRESH SPINACH**
½ **TEASPOON GROUND SALT**
⅛ **TEASPOON GROUND BLACK PEPPER**
4 **LARGE EGGS**

Makes 2 servings
241 calories per serving

Preheat the oven to 400°F.

Cook the onion in the olive oil in a skillet over medium heat, stirring, until softened, about 5 minutes. Add the spinach and cover, stirring occasionally. Cook until the spinach is wilted, 2 to 3 minutes. Add the salt and pepper and cook for 2 more minutes.

In a small bowl whisk the eggs. Place the eggs in a small baking dish. Gently place the spinach mixture on top of the eggs. Bake for 15 minutes, or until the eggs are cooked through. Cut and serve.

SALADS

Citrus-Coriander Grilled Chicken and Quinoa Tabbouleh

---

1 EACH LEMON, LIME, AND ORANGE, ZESTED
  AND JUICED
½ CUP EXTRA VIRGIN OLIVE OIL
1 TEASPOON GROUND CORIANDER
1 TEASPOON GROUND CLOVES
PINCH OF GROUND CINNAMON
4 CHICKEN BREAST HALVES, SKINLESS AND
  BONELESS
1½ CUPS QUINOA
½ TEASPOON SALT
8 OUNCES FRESH PARSLEY, FINELY MINCED
4 OUNCES FRESH MINT, FINELY MINCED
2 TOMATOES, SEEDED AND DICED
1 BUNCH SCALLIONS, CUT ON THE BIAS
GROUND BLACK PEPPER
CHOPPED SCALLIONS FOR GARNISH

Makes 4 servings
488 calories per serving

In a mixing bowl, mix together half of the citrus juices, ¼ cup of the olive oil, and the coriander, cloves, and cinnamon. Whisk together all the marinade ingredients and pour over the chicken breasts.

Place the quinoa in a strainer. Rinse under cold running water until the water runs clear; drain. Mix the quinoa, the citrus zest, 2 cups water, and the salt in a heavy medium saucepan. Bring to a boil. Reduce the heat to medium-low, cover, and simmer until the quinoa is just tender and almost all the water is absorbed, about 20 minutes. Drain. Mix in the remaining ¼ cup olive oil and the remaining citrus juice, and the parsley, mint, tomatoes, and scallions with the quinoa, and fold all the ingredients together. Season to taste with salt and pepper, possibly adding a bit more lemon juice.

Remove the chicken from the marinade and grill for 4 to 6 minutes per side, or until done in the center.

Place the tabbouleh salad in the center of four plates. Slice the chicken breasts at an angle, creating medallions, and fan out across the top of the tabbouleh. Sprinkle the top with a few chopped scallions for color.

Israeli Salad

4 TOMATOES, CHOPPED
1 CUCUMBER, PEELED, SEEDED, AND CHOPPED
½ CUP FINELY CHOPPED FRESH SPINACH
1 TABLESPOON CRUMBLED FETA CHEESE
1 TABLESPOON FRESH LEMON JUICE
1 TABLESPOON OLIVE OIL
CHOPPED FRESH MINT TO TASTE*

Makes 2 servings
150 calories per serving

Toss the tomatoes, cucumber, spinach, and feta cheese in a medium bowl. Set aside.

In a small bowl mix the lemon juice and olive oil. Mix well. Drizzle the dressing onto the salad, add fresh mint, and serve.

Orange and Mushroom Spinach Salad

Dressing

1 CUP FRESH ORANGE JUICE
3 TABLESPOONS MINCED GARLIC
¼ CUP OLIVE OIL
½ CUP BALSAMIC VINEGAR OR
    RED WINE VINEGAR

Makes 8 servings
100 calories per serving

Salad

4 ORANGES, PEELED AND WHITE PITH REMOVED
2 CUPS STEMMED FRESH SPINACH
2 CUPS CHOPPED MUSHROOMS
1 CUP CHOPPED CUCUMBER
2 TOMATOES, COARSELY CHOPPED

Makes 8 servings
180 calories per serving

For the dressing

In a small bowl, whisk together all the ingredients. Set aside.

For the salad

Cut the oranges into small segments. Place in a large bowl. Tear the spinach and place in the bowl; add the mushrooms, cucumber, and tomatoes. Toss well.

Warm the dressing in a small pot over low heat. Stir frequently until the dressing is warm, 4 to 5 minutes. Pour evenly over the salad. Toss for a few minutes so that the dressing is evenly distributed throughout the salad. Serve warm or cold.

Orange Tuna Spinach Salad

2 ORANGES, ZESTED AND JUICED
¼ CUP HONEY
¼ CUP OLIVE OIL
SALT
GROUND BLACK PEPPER
4 TUNA FILLETS
1 POUND FRESH SPINACH, WASHED AND
    STEMMED
1 RED ONION, THINLY SLICED
1 ENGLISH CUCUMBER, PEELED,
    SLICED IN HALF LENGTHWISE, AND
    THINLY SLICED INTO HALF ROUNDS
1 TOMATO, SLICED INTO WEDGES

Makes 4 servings
408 calories per serving

Whisk together the orange juice, honey, olive oil, and salt and pepper to taste. Pour half of the dressing over the tuna along with the orange zest. Marinate the tuna for 1 hour. Grill or sauté the tuna for 4 to 6 minutes on each side, until thoroughly cooked in the center.

Toss the spinach, red onion, and cucumber with the remaining dressing. Place the tossed spinach greens, onion, and cucumber on a plate. Place the cooked tuna in the middle of the spinach. Garnish around the tuna with the tomato wedges and garnish the top of the tuna with a thinly sliced orange wheel.

Note: Salmon also works well with this recipe.

Herbed Quinoa

1½ CUPS QUINOA
1 TEASPOON DRIED THYME (SEE NOTE)
1 TEASPOON DRIED ROSEMARY (SEE NOTE)
1 TEASPOON DRIED OREGANO (SEE NOTE)
2½ TABLESPOONS EXTRA VIRGIN OLIVE OIL

Makes 2 servings
342 calories per serving

Cook the quinoa in a large saucepan of boiling water for 10 minutes. Drain in a sieve and rinse under cold water. Gently stir the herbs, if desired, and the olive oil into the quinoa. Set the sieve with the quinoa over a saucepan filled with 1½ inches boiling water (the sieve should not touch the water) and steam the quinoa, covered with a lid, until fluffy and dry, 10 to 12 minutes. (Check the water level in the pan occasionally, adding more water if necessary.)

Note: If you do not use herbs, simply steam the quinoa with the olive oil until fluffy.

Quinoa Salad with Garbanzo Beans, Feta, and Tomatoes

1 CUP QUINOA
ONE 15½-OUNCE CAN GARBANZO BEANS (CHICKPEAS), RINSED AND DRAINED
1 CUP DICED TOMATOES
½ CUP CRUMBLED FETA CHEESE
½ CUP CHOPPED ONIONS
3 TABLESPOONS FRESH LEMON JUICE
1½ TABLESPOONS OLIVE OIL
2 TEASPOONS GRATED LEMON ZEST
1 TEASPOON SALT
GROUND BLACK PEPPER

Makes 3 servings
423 calories per serving

Cook the quinoa in 2 cups boiling water for 10 minutes. Drain and put the quinoa in a covered bowl; set aside for 10 minutes. Transfer the quinoa to a large bowl; let cool. Mix in the remaining ingredients. Season with salt and pepper and serve.

Toasted Quinoa Salad with Red Bell Pepper and Mushrooms

½ CUP QUINOA

2 CUPS CHICKEN OR VEGETABLE BROTH

1 RED BELL PEPPER, CHOPPED

24 LARGE SPINACH LEAVES OR 6 CUPS FROZEN SPINACH, COOKED

2 CUPS STEMMED AND CHOPPED MUSHROOMS

2 TABLESPOONS OLIVE OIL

2 LARGE TOMATOES, SEEDED AND CHOPPED

1 CUP CHOPPED CUCUMBER

2½ TABLESPOONS FRESH LEMON JUICE

Makes 3 servings

278 calories per serving

Place the quinoa in a heavy, large saucepan with the broth. Cook over medium heat until broth boils. Reduce the heat to medium-low, cover, and simmer until the quinoa is fluffy and the broth is absorbed, approximately 15 minutes. Uncover and let the quinoa cool.

Place the red bell pepper, spinach, and mushrooms in a medium skillet over medium-low heat. Drizzle with 1 tablespoon of the olive oil. Lightly sauté for 10 minutes. Add the quinoa and sauté for another 5 minutes, or until the quinoa is slightly browned.

In a large bowl combine the quinoa, red bell pepper, spinach, mushrooms, tomatoes, cucumber, lemon juice, and the remaining 1 tablespoon of olive oil. Toss the salad and serve.

Cucumber, Tomato, and Pita Salad

1 WHOLE-WHEAT PITA

OLIVE OIL TO DRIZZLE

2 CUCUMBERS, PEELED, SEEDED, AND CHOPPED

3 TOMATOES, CHOPPED

1 TABLESPOON OLIVE OIL

1 TABLESPOON FRESH LEMON JUICE

1 TEASPOON LEMON ZEST

1 ORANGE, PEELED AND CHOPPED

1 TABLESPOON BALSAMIC VINEGAR*

Makes 2 servings

261 calories per serving

Preheat the oven to 375°F. Cut up the pita into thin strips and lightly drizzle with olive oil. Place evenly across a baking sheet. Bake for 10 minutes, or until lightly browned.

Combine the cucumbers, tomatoes, olive oil, lemon juice and zest, and the orange in a medium bowl. Mix in the pita strips. For extra flavor add balsamic vinegar, if desired.

Tuna and Garbanzo Bean Salad

1 GARLIC CLOVE, MINCED
3 TABLESPOONS FRESH LEMON JUICE
½ TEASPOON BLACK PEPPER
¼ CUP EXTRA VIRGIN OLIVE OIL
ONE 15½-OUNCE CAN GARBANZO BEANS
   (CHICKPEAS), RINSED AND DRAINED
3 TOMATOES, CUT INTO PIECES
1 CUCUMBER, PEELED, SEEDED, AND DICED
TWO 6-OUNCE CANS TUNA IN WATER*

Makes 3 servings
420 calories per serving

Whisk together the garlic, lemon juice, and pepper in a small bowl, then add the oil in a slow stream, whisking until well combined. Set aside for 10 minutes.

In a medium bowl combine the garbanzo beans, tomatoes, and cucumber. Toss gently and add half of the dressing. Transfer to a larger bowl, adding the tuna and the remaining dressing. Toss gently.

Spinach Salad with Red Onions and Orange and Hummus Dressing

2 TABLESPOONS HUMMUS (RECIPE PAGE 215 OR
   STORE-BOUGHT)
1 TABLESPOON FRESH ORANGE JUICE
1 TEASPOON GRATED ORANGE ZEST
2 RED ONIONS, CHOPPED
4 CUPS CHOPPED FRESH SPINACH
1 CUP CHOPPED CUCUMBER

Makes 3 servings
125 calories per serving

In a small bowl mix the hummus, orange juice, and orange zest. Set aside.

In a large bowl combine the onions, spinach, and cucumber. Slowly add the hummus-orange dressing.

Toss well and serve.

Quinoa Tabbouleh with Avocados and Feta Cheese

½ **CUP QUINOA**
2 **CUPS CHOPPED TOMATOES**
1 **CUCUMBER, PEELED, SEEDED, AND FINELY CHOPPED**
1 **CUP CHOPPED FRESH ITALIAN PARSLEY***
4 **GREEN ONIONS, CHOPPED***
½ **CUP CRUMBLED FETA CHEESE**
¼ **CUP CHOPPED FRESH MINT***
1 **TABLESPOON GRATED LEMON ZEST**
6 **TABLESPOONS OLIVE OIL**
3 **TABLESPOONS FRESH LEMON JUICE**
2 **AVOCADOS, PEELED, PITTED, AND SLICED**

Makes 3 servings
450 calories per serving

Boil the quinoa in 1½ cups water. Cook for 10 minutes and then simmer for another 10 minutes, or until the liquid is absorbed.

In a large bowl combine the tomatoes, cucumber, parsley (optional), green onions (optional), feta cheese, mint (optional), and lemon zest. Once the quinoa is cool, add it to the mixture. Sprinkle with the olive oil and lemon juice. Stir well. Add the avocado slices before serving.

Baked Mushrooms and Feta

12 **MUSHROOMS, STEMMED**
2 **CUPS CHOPPED FRESH SPINACH OR 1 CUP FROZEN SPINACH, THAWED WITH WATER SQUEEZED OUT**
1 **TABLESPOON OLIVE OIL**
3 **TABLESPOONS CRUMBLED FETA CHEESE**

Makes 2 servings
150 calories per serving

Preheat the oven to 375°F. Place the mushrooms, rounded side down, on a baking sheet. Heat in the oven for 10 minutes, or until warm. While the mushrooms are cooking, sauté the spinach over medium-high heat in the olive oil until the spinach is wilted. Remove the spinach from the pan and place it in a small bowl. Mix in the feta cheese.

Place the mushrooms on a large plate and place 1 spoonful of the spinach-feta mixture in the center of each mushroom.

SOUPS

Roasted Tomato Soup with Garlic

3½ POUNDS TOMATOES, CUT LENGTHWISE
GROUND BLACK PEPPER
7 TABLESPOONS OLIVE OIL
¼ CUP MINCED GARLIC
1½ TEASPOONS DRIED ROSEMARY*
1½ TEASPOONS DRIED THYME*
6 CUPS LOW-SODIUM CHICKEN BROTH

Makes 4 servings
329 calories per serving

Preheat the oven to 400°F. Place the tomatoes, cut side up, in a baking pan. Sprinkle lightly with black pepper. Drizzle the tomatoes with 4 tablespoons of the olive oil. Roast until the tomatoes are brown and tender, about 1 hour. Let cool slightly.

Transfer the tomatoes and any juices to a food processor. Process until slightly chunky by pulsating the on/off switch. Heat the remaining 3 tablespoons oil in a large pot over medium-high heat. Add the garlic and sauté for 2 to 3 minutes. Stir in the tomatoes and the herbs (optional). Add the chicken broth; bring to a boil. Reduce the heat and simmer until the soup thickens slightly, about 25 minutes. Serve hot or let cool in the refrigerator for 30 minutes before serving.

Spicy Cucumber-Avocado Soup

1 AVOCADO, PEELED, PITTED, AND ½ CHOPPED
1–2 CUCUMBERS, PEELED, SEEDED, AND DICED
1 CUP SMALL ICE CUBES
1 TEASPOON FRESH LEMON OR LIME JUICE
1 TEASPOON SALT, OR TO TASTE
1 CUP NONFAT YOGURT FOR A SMOOTHER
   CONSISTENCY*
3 TABLESPOONS CHOPPED FRESH CHIVES*

Blend the unchopped half of the avocado, the cucumbers, ice cubes, lemon juice, salt, and yogurt (optional) in a food processor. Garnish with the chopped avocado and chives, if desired.

Makes 2 servings
251 calories per serving

Summer Garden Gazpacho

2 TOMATOES, SEEDED AND CHOPPED
3 TABLESPOONS OLIVE OIL
1 GARLIC CLOVE, CHOPPED
3 CUPS FRESH TOMATO JUICE, OR CHILLED
   REGULAR OR SPICY MIXED VEGETABLE JUICE
1 CUP CANNED GARBANZO BEANS (CHICKPEAS),
   RINSED AND DRAINED
1 RED BELL PEPPER, CHOPPED
1 CUP CHOPPED CUCUMBER
GROUND BLACK PEPPER

Place the tomatoes, olive oil, and garlic in a food processor and blend until a coarse purée forms. While processing, gradually add the tomato juice or vegetable juice and process until smooth. Transfer the mixture to a medium bowl. Mix in the garbanzo beans, red bell pepper, and cucumber. Season the soup with black pepper.

Makes 3 servings
295 calories per serving

Garlic Soup with Tomatoes

3 TOMATOES, CHOPPED
10 GARLIC CLOVES, PEELED AND COARSELY
     CHOPPED
3 RED BELL PEPPERS, CUT INTO CHUNKS
½ CUP OLIVE OIL
GROUND BLACK PEPPER

Makes 3 servings
386 calories per serving

In a food processor, pulse the tomatoes, half of the chopped garlic, and the red bell peppers until coarsely chopped.

In a medium saucepan, heat the olive oil over medium heat. Add the tomato, garlic, and red bell pepper mixture to the pan. Cook for 5 minutes, stirring frequently. Stir in the remaining garlic and 1¾ cups water. Bring to a boil. Lower the heat and simmer for 10 minutes. Season with black pepper. Serve hot or let cool in the refrigerator for 30 minutes prior to serving.

Roasted Tomato and Red Bell Pepper Soup

2¼ POUNDS TOMATOES, HALVED LENGTHWISE
2 LARGE RED BELL PEPPERS, QUARTERED
1 ONION, COARSELY CHOPPED
4 LARGE GARLIC CLOVES, PEELED
2 TABLESPOONS OLIVE OIL
GROUND BLACK PEPPER

Makes 3 servings
211 calories per serving

Preheat the oven to 450°F. Arrange the tomatoes (cut side up), red bell peppers, onion, and garlic in a large baking pan. Drizzle with the oil and sprinkle generously with black pepper. Roast the vegetables until brown and tender, approximately 45 minutes. Turn the red bell peppers and onion occasionally, approximately every 10 minutes. Remove from the oven. Set aside and let cool.

Transfer the vegetables and any juices to a food processor. Purée the vegetables. Slowly add spoonfuls of water (about 2 cups) until the soup is the desired consistency. Chill until cold, about 2 hours.

Chicken, Spinach, and Quinoa Soup

2 TABLESPOONS OLIVE OIL

4 CHICKEN BREAST HALVES, SKINLESS AND BONELESS

1 LARGE ONION, COARSELY CHOPPED

2 LARGE GARLIC CLOVES, MINCED

4 QUARTS WATER

2 CUPS LOW-SODIUM CHICKEN BROTH

1½ CUPS SLICED RED BELL PEPPERS

1 POUND FRESH SPINACH, WASHED, STEMMED, AND CHOPPED

½ CUP QUINOA

GROUND BLACK PEPPER

½ TEASPOON CRUMBLED DRIED MINT*

½ TEASPOON CRUMBLED DRIED ROSEMARY*

Makes 4 servings

312 calories per serving

In a stockpot heat the oil over moderately high heat. Lower the heat to medium, add the chicken and cook, turning the chicken occasionally. Once the chicken is completely cooked, approximately 20 minutes, remove and set aside to cool.

In the same pot combine the onion and garlic and cook, stirring, for 10 minutes, or until the onion is golden. Add the water and the broth, and bring the liquid to a boil, skimming the froth; simmer the mixture, uncovered, for 2 hours.

In the meantime, cut the chicken breasts into 1½-inch pieces. Add the red bell peppers, the chicken, and the spinach to the broth; bring the liquid to a boil; and add the quinoa. Boil the soup, stirring, for 10 minutes, or until the quinoa is tender, and season it with black pepper. Sprinkle with herbs, if desired.

MAIN DISHES

Lemon Chicken

¼ **CUP FRESH LEMON JUICE**

3 **TABLESPOONS MINCED GARLIC**

2 **TABLESPOONS KOSHER SALT**

2 **TEASPOONS GROUND BLACK PEPPER**

½ **CUP OLIVE OIL**

12 **WHOLE CHICKEN LEGS, SKINLESS**

8 **CHICKEN BREAST HALVES, SKINLESS AND BONELESS**

6 **LEMONS, CUT CROSSWISE INTO ½-INCH-THICK SLICES**

Makes 8 servings
474 calories per serving

Preheat the oven to 325°F. Whisk together the lemon juice, garlic, ½ tablespoon of the salt, and ½ teaspoon of the pepper in a large bowl. As you whisk the ingredients together, add the oil, slowly, to the mix. Set aside.

Coat the bottom of a lasagna-style baking pan with some of the above mixture. Place the chicken evenly across the pan. Drizzle the remaining mixture and salt and pepper until the chicken is fully coated. Turn the chicken over if necessary to ensure that it is entirely covered. Place the lemon slices throughout the pan.

Place the pan in the center of the oven. Bake 30 minutes, or until the chicken is cooked through.

Orange-Marinated Tuna Kebabs

1½ **POUNDS TUNA STEAKS, CUT INTO SIXTEEN 1- TO 1¼-INCH CUBES**

10 TOMATO CHUNKS OR CHERRY TOMATOES

8 MUSHROOMS, STEMMED

EIGHT 8- TO 10-INCH WOODEN SKEWERS, SOAKED IN WATER 30 MINUTES

1 TABLESPOON OLIVE OIL

2 TEASPOONS MINCED GARLIC

1¾ TEASPOONS GRATED ORANGE ZEST

1½ TEASPOONS MINCED FRESH ROSEMARY*

Makes 4 servings

195 calories per serving

Preheat the oven to 375°F. Place the tuna, tomatoes, and mushrooms on the skewers. Set aside. In a small bowl mix the olive oil, garlic, and orange zest. Stir in rosemary, if desired. Brush the skewers with the orange dressing. Make sure that you coat all sides of the skewers. (You may also marinate the skewers for 24 hours in the orange dressing prior to cooking.)

Place the skewers on a baking sheet covered with aluminum foil. Place in the oven and cook for 20 minutes, or until the tuna is cooked through, rotating occasionally.

Note: This recipe can be prepared either on the grill or in the oven.

Chicken Breasts Stuffed with Feta Cheese and Spinach

Spinach and Feta Cheese Filling

2 TABLESPOONS EXTRA VIRGIN OLIVE OIL

1 LARGE GARLIC CLOVE, MINCED

¼ CUP CHICKEN BROTH OR WATER

2 POUNDS FRESH SPINACH, WASHED AND
    STEMMED

COARSE SALT AND FRESHLY GROUND
    BLACK PEPPER TO TASTE

½ CUP CRUMBLED FETA CHEESE

4 LARGE CHICKEN BREAST HALVES,
    SKINLESS AND BONELESS

Makes 4 servings

254 calories per serving

Preheat the oven to 350°F. Heat the oil in a pan over medium heat. Add the garlic and cook for 15 to 20 seconds. Add the chicken broth and immediately put the spinach in. Cook for 2 minutes, stirring frequently. Season with salt and pepper. Set aside in a shallow lasagna pan to cool. When cool, gently stir in the feta cheese.

Place a chicken breast on the work surface. Pound gently until the chicken breast is ½ inch thick. Place a few spoonfuls of the feta cheese filling on one side of the chicken breast. Fold the chicken breast in half. Repeat with each remaining chicken breast.

Lightly coat a large baking pan with olive oil. Place the chicken breasts in the pan, side by side. Bake until the chicken is thoroughly cooked, approximately 30 minutes.

Note: Goat cheese is also delicious in this recipe.

Open-Faced Hummus and Spinach Sandwich

1 WHOLE-WHEAT PITA
2 TABLESPOONS HUMMUS
   (RECIPE PAGE 215 OR STORE-BOUGHT)
1 TOMATO, SLICED
½ CUCUMBER, PEELED AND SLICED
5 FRESH SPINACH LEAVES, STEMMED
2 MUSHROOMS, STEMMED AND SLICED
¼ RED BELL PEPPER, SLICED LENGTHWISE
½ AVOCADO, PEELED, PITTED, AND SLICED*

Makes 1 serving
247 calories per serving without avocado, 407 with avocado

Cut the pita so that you are only using one round half. Spread the hummus on the pita. Layer the tomato, cucumber, spinach leaves, mushrooms, red bell pepper, and avocado, if desired. Fold the pita in half or eat open-faced.

Tuna in Tomato Sauce

⅓ CUP EXTRA VIRGIN OLIVE OIL
2 TABLESPOONS MINCED GARLIC
½ TEASPOON PAPRIKA*
⅛ TEASPOON CAYENNE PEPPER*
12 TOMATOES, CHOPPED
   (RESERVE JUICE FOR SAUCE)
ONE 1½-POUND PIECE TUNA OR ANY WHITE FISH,
   CUT CROSSWISE INTO ½-INCH-THICK PIECES
SALT
GROUND BLACK PEPPER

Makes 3 servings
480 calories per serving

Heat the oil in a large saucepan over medium-high heat. Add the garlic and cook for 1 minute, or until brown. Add the spices (optional) and cook for about 30 seconds, stirring occasionally. Stir in the tomatoes (including the juice) and simmer, uncovered, stirring occasionally, for 20 to 25 minutes.

Season the tuna with salt and pepper and arrange on top of the sauce. Cook, covered, until the fish is thoroughly cooked, 5 to 10 minutes depending on the thickness of the fish. Place the fish on a plate and cover with the sauce.

Chicken Burgers

2 WHOLE-WHEAT PITAS
1 TABLESPOON OLIVE OIL
2 CHICKEN BREAST HALVES,
    SKINLESS AND BONELESS
1 TOMATO, CHOPPED
1 AVOCADO, PEELED, PITTED, AND CHOPPED
2 TABLESPOONS CRUMBLED FETA CHEESE*
8 FRESH SPINACH LEAVES, STEMMED
½ RED BELL PEPPER, CUT LENGTHWISE

*Makes 4 servings
260 calories per serving*

Cut the pitas into halves so that you can open them up and use them as buns. Set aside.

In a medium pan heat the oil over medium heat. Add the chicken and cook for 20 minutes, or until browned, turning the chicken occasionally. Set aside and let cool. Cut the chicken into at least 6 strips per breast.

In a small bowl mix the tomato, avocado, and feta cheese, if desired.

Open up half a pita and add 3 chicken strips, 2 spinach leaves, a few red bell pepper strips, and a few spoonfuls of the tomato mixture. Repeat with each pita half.

Sautéed Chicken with Peppers and Avocado Salsa

2 WHOLE-WHEAT PITAS, CUT INTO SMALL STRIPS
¼ CUP DICED AVOCADO
¼ CUP CHOPPED ONION
1 TABLESPOON FRESH LEMON JUICE
2 TABLESPOONS OLIVE OIL
¼ CUP NONFAT YOGURT*
3 CHICKEN BREAST HALVES, SKINLESS AND
    BONELESS, CUT INTO STRIPS
3 RED BELL PEPPERS, CUT LENGTHWISE INTO
    STRIPS
¼ CUP CHOPPED FRESH CILANTRO*

*Makes 4 servings
406 calories per serving*

Preheat the oven to 350°F. Wrap the whole wheat pita strips in aluminum foil and heat in the oven for 20 minutes, or until crisp.

In the meantime, combine the avocado, onion, lemon juice, 1 tablespoon of the olive oil, and yogurt (optional) in a small bowl. Set aside.

Heat the remaining oil in a large nonstick skillet over high heat. Add the chicken and red bell peppers to the skillet; sauté until the chicken is cooked through, about 8 minutes. In a large bowl mix together the chicken, red bell peppers, and pita strips. Place on plates and top with the avocado mixture and cilantro, if using.

Lemon and Garlic Roast Chicken

10 VERY THIN LEMON SLICES, SEEDED
**4 CHICKEN BREAST HALVES,
    SKINLESS AND BONELESS**
4 TEASPOONS FRESH LEMON JUICE
2 GARLIC CLOVES, COARSELY CHOPPED
GROUND BLACK PEPPER
1 CUP CANNED LOW-SODIUM CHICKEN BROTH

Makes 4 servings
142 calories per serving

Preheat the oven to 450°F. Place the lemon slices evenly across the chicken breast halves. Place the chicken in a large baking pan and drizzle 1 teaspoon lemon juice over each breast; sprinkle with the garlic and black pepper. Pour ½ cup of the broth around the chicken.

Roast the chicken until brown and cooked through, basting once or twice with the pan juices, about 30 minutes.

Place the juices from the pan and the remaining ½ cup broth in a small pot and simmer on medium-low for 15 minutes. When ready to serve, pour the juice mixture over the chicken.

Grilled Tomato and Feta Sandwiches

2 WHOLE-WHEAT PITAS
2 TABLESPOONS OLIVE OIL
4 LARGE GARLIC CLOVES, FINELY CHOPPED
¾ CUP CRUMBLED FETA CHEESE
**2 LARGE TOMATOES, THINLY
    SLICED INTO ROUNDS**
½ ONION, THINLY SLICED
**1 TABLESPOON CHOPPED MIXED FRESH HERBS
    (TARRAGON, THYME, AND ROSEMARY)***

Makes 2 servings
496 calories per serving

Warm the pitas in a toaster oven or bake in a preheated 370°F oven for 5 minutes on a baking sheet. In a small bowl mix the olive oil, garlic, and feta cheese. Cut the pitas in half and coat the insides with the cheese mixture. Bake in the oven for another 3 minutes. Add the tomatoes and onion to the insides of the pitas. Sprinkle with herbs, if desired, and serve.

Note: Goat cheese is also delicious in this recipe.

Vegetable Pita Pizzas

2 WHOLE-WHEAT PITAS

3 TABLESPOONS OLIVE OIL PLUS ADDITIONAL
   FOR BRUSHING THE PITA ROUNDS

1⅓ CUPS CRUMBLED FETA CHEESE
   OR GRATED MOZZARELLA

1 RED ONION, THINLY SLICED

6 MUSHROOMS, STEMMED AND SLICED

2 GARLIC CLOVES, MINCED

1 RED BELL PEPPER, THINLY SLICED

½ CUP COARSELY CHOPPED FRESH SPINACH

1 CUP CHOPPED TOMATOES

Makes 4 servings
336 calories per serving

Preheat the oven to 350°F. Halve the pitas, forming 4 rounds, and place on a baking sheet with the rough sides up. Brush the tops lightly with olive oil. Toast the rounds until they are slightly browned, approximately 5 minutes. Sprinkle 1 cup of the feta cheese evenly onto the rounds and bake for 1 more minute.

In the meantime, sauté the onion, mushrooms, and garlic in the 3 tablespoons olive oil over medium-high heat. Add the red bell pepper and spinach, and sauté for 5 more minutes, stirring frequently. Top the rounds with the vegetables. Add the tomatoes and the remaining ⅓ cup feta cheese. Bake the pita pizzas for 5 minutes.

SNACKS AND SIDES

Tomato and Feta Galette

½ CUP OLIVE OIL
3 TO 4 GARLIC CLOVES, PEELED
4 WHOLE-WHEAT PITAS
2 TOMATOES, SLICED
SALT
GROUND BLACK PEPPER
1 CUP CRUMBLED FETA CHEESE

Makes 4 servings
525 calories per serving

Preheat the oven to 350°F. In a small pot, heat the olive oil and garlic over medium heat just until the garlic turns brown. Remove from the heat and strain the garlic out of the hot oil. Set the oil aside to cool.

Lay the whole pitas on a baking sheet. Brush the pitas with the garlic olive oil. Place 2 to 3 tomato slices on each pita. Season the tomatoes with salt and pepper, if desired, and sprinkle the feta cheese over the top of the tomatoes. Bake in the oven for 6 to 8 minutes, until the cheese is hot.

Garbanzo Bean and Feta Pitas

ONE 15½-OUNCE CAN GARBANZO BEANS
    (CHICKPEAS), RINSED AND DRAINED
½ CUP OLIVE OIL
1½ CUPS COARSELY CHOPPED TOMATOES
1½ CUPS COARSELY CHOPPED CUCUMBERS
1 CUP COARSELY CRUMBLED FETA CHEESE
½ CUP CHOPPED RED ONIONS
SALT
GROUND BLACK PEPPER
½ CUP NONFAT YOGURT*
2 WHOLE-WHEAT PITAS, HALVED CROSSWISE

Makes 4 servings
574 calories per serving

Place the drained garbanzo beans in a medium bowl. Mix in the olive oil.

Add the tomatoes, cucumbers, feta cheese, and red onions to the garbanzo beans. Season the bean salad to taste with salt and pepper. Mix in the yogurt, if desired. Fill the pita halves with the bean salad. Serve immediately.

Pita Chips with Garbanzo Bean–Cumin Dip

2 WHOLE-WHEAT PITAS

1 TABLESPOON EXTRA VIRGIN OLIVE OIL PLUS ADDITIONAL OIL FOR SPRINKLING THE PITA WEDGES

2 TEASPOONS GROUND CUMIN

ONE 15½-OUNCE CAN GARBANZO BEANS (CHICKPEAS), DRAINED, LIQUID RESERVED

3 TABLESPOONS FRESH LEMON JUICE

1 SMALL GARLIC CLOVE, PEELED

2 TABLESPOONS FINELY CHOPPED RED BELL PEPPER

Makes 4 servings
260 calories per serving

Preheat the oven to 350°F. Cut each whole-wheat pita bread round into triangular wedges. Place the pita wedges in a single layer on a baking sheet. Sprinkle with olive oil. Bake until the wedges are crisp and golden, about 10 minutes. Let cool completely.

Stir the cumin in a small dry skillet over medium-low heat for about 30 seconds. Remove from the heat. Combine the garbanzo beans, ¼ cup of the reserved garbanzo bean liquid, the lemon juice, 1 tablespoon oil, and the garlic, red bell pepper, and cumin in a food processor. Purée until smooth. For a smoother consistency add more garbanzo bean liquid.

Serve in a bowl with the pita chips.

Tuna in Avocado Halves

ONE 6-OUNCE CAN TUNA IN WATER

1 TABLESPOON OLIVE OIL

1 TEASPOON FRESH LEMON JUICE

2 TABLESPOONS BALSAMIC VINEGAR*

1 AVOCADO

Makes 2 servings
321 calories per serving

Drain the tuna and set aside. In a small bowl whisk together the olive oil, lemon juice, and vinegar (optional). Halve and pit the avocado. Fill the halves with tuna and drizzle with the dressing.

Sautéed Mixed Mushrooms

½ **CUP OLIVE OIL**
3 **POUNDS MUSHROOMS, STEMS AND CAPS SEPARATED**
1 **TEASPOON FRESH LEMON JUICE**
1 **TEASPOON SALT**
½ **TEASPOON GROUND BLACK PEPPER**
1 **TABLESPOON FINELY CHOPPED GARLIC**

Makes 5 servings
218 calories per serving

Heat olive oil in a large skillet over medium-high heat. Sauté the mushrooms with the lemon juice and a pinch of salt and pepper, stirring occasionally, until the mushrooms are tender. Add in the garlic and the remaining salt and pepper. Sauté for another 2 minutes. This dish makes a great complement to any chicken or fish entrée.

Avocado and Chicken in Tomato Cups

1 **TABLESPOON EXTRA VIRGIN OLIVE OIL**
⅓ **CUP MINCED ONION**
1 **LARGE GARLIC CLOVE, MINCED**
½ **CUP BOILED AND CHOPPED CHICKEN (1 SKINLESS AND BONELESS CHICKEN BREAST)**
1 **AVOCADO, PEELED, PITTED, AND CHOPPED**
3 **TABLESPOONS FRESH LEMON JUICE**
12 **VINE-RIPENED TOMATOES**
3 **TABLESPOONS CRUMBLED FETA CHEESE**

Makes 6 servings
130 calories per serving

Preheat the oven to 350°F. Heat the oil in a medium skillet over medium-high heat. Add the onion and garlic. Sauté for 3 minutes, or until the onion and garlic are browned. Reduce the heat slightly and add the chopped chicken. Sauté for another 3 minutes. Place the ingredients in a medium bowl and add the avocado and lemon juice. Mix well and set aside.

Cut the tomatoes into halves and scoop out the centers. Place spoonfuls of the chicken-avocado mixture in the tomatoes. Place the stuffed tomatoes in a large baking pan. Sprinkle the tops of the tomatoes with the feta cheese. Bake for 10 minutes.

Note: Goat cheese is also delicious in this recipe.

Lemon-Glazed Vegetables

3 CUPS COARSELY CHOPPED FRESH SPINACH

1 ONION, CHOPPED

**2 CUPS STEMMED AND CHOPPED MUSHROOMS
(SEE NOTE)**

2 TABLESPOONS OLIVE OIL

3 TABLESPOONS FRESH LEMON JUICE

**3 TABLESPOONS GRATED LEMON ZEST, PLUS
ADDITIONAL TO TASTE**

Makes 2 servings
188 calories per serving

Preheat the oven to 375°F. In a large baking pan place all the vegetables and ¾ cup water. Drizzle lightly with the olive oil, 1 tablespoon of the lemon juice, and 1 teaspoon of the lemon zest. Toss gently before cooking. Cook for 10 minutes, stirring the vegetables occasionally. Remove the pan from the oven and add the remaining 2 tablespoons lemon juice and 2 tablespoons plus 2 teaspoons zest. Cook for another 10 minutes, stirring occasionally. Add additional lemon zest to taste, if desired.

Note: You may add any vegetables you like to this recipe.

DIPS AND DRESSINGS

Hummus

TWO 15 ½-OUNCE CANS GARBANZO BEANS
    (CHICKPEAS), RINSED AND DRAINED
4 GARLIC CLOVES, MINCED
⅔ CUP TAHINI
¼ CUP FRESH LEMON JUICE, OR TO TASTE
¼ CUP OLIVE OIL, OR TO TASTE

Makes 10 to 12 servings
312 calories per serving

In a food processor purée the garbanzo beans with the garlic, tahini (stir well prior to adding), lemon juice, oil, and ½ cup water until the hummus is smooth. Stop the processor occasionally to scrape the hummus off the sides. Add water, if necessary, to thin the hummus to the desired consistency, and transfer the hummus to a bowl. Cover and store in the refrigerator.

Hummus is a perfect dip for both vegetables and whole-wheat pita chips.

Guacamole

2 PLUM TOMATOES
2 FIRM-RIPE AVOCADOS, PEELED, PITTED,
    AND CHOPPED
2 TABLESPOONS MINCED RED ONION
3 TABLESPOONS FRESH LEMON OR LIME JUICE,
    PLUS MORE TO TASTE
1 TEASPOON MINCED GARLIC, PLUS
    MORE TO TASTE

Makes 4 servings
175 calories per serving

Cut the tomatoes into halves. Scrape out the seeds. In a food processor combine the tomatoes, avocados, onion, lemon juice, and garlic. Blend until smooth with small avocado chunks. Add more lemon juice and garlic to taste, if desired.

Homemade guacamole is fantastic as a dip or as a salad dressing.

Tomato Salsa

1 CUP DICED TOMATOES
3 TABLESPOONS CHOPPED ONION
2 TABLESPOONS FRESH LEMON OR LIME JUICE
¼ CUP CHOPPED FRESH CILANTRO*

Makes 2 servings
29 calories per serving

Place all the ingredients in a food processor. Blend, using the on/off switch, until the salsa is smooth chunky.

Tomato salsa is perfect as a dip or as a salad dressing.

BOOTCAMP360 SUCCESS STORY

RECRUIT SARA STAYING FIT FOREVER

"It is now about choosing and maintaining a healthy lifestyle for both of us."

PRE-WEDDING: 175 LBS. BODY FAT: 23%

WEDDING DAY: 155 LBS. BODY FAT: 21%

TODAY: 148 LBS. BODY FAT: 18.5%

SOMETHING OLD **SOMETHING NEW** **SOMETHING FOREVER**

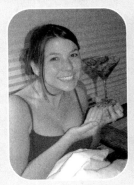 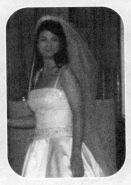 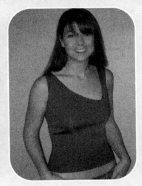

At five feet eleven inches, I suppose I should count myself lucky to have more body surface area than the average woman, over which I can spread the occasional extra pound or two. But two happy years into my marriage, it's still a challenge to stay committed to being fit after the honeymoon is over. My husband and I find that we are busier than ever, between my full-time career and his full-time graduate school curriculum. And I thought planning a wedding took a lot out of me! We literally have to schedule dates just to make enough time for each other—not to mention making time to exercise and stay fit.

Although blissful in most aspects, I can't say my first year of marriage was easy from a fitness standpoint. Once the honeymoon was over, life did eventually go back to normal, and without the wedding date hanging over my head as a target, it was tempting to fall back into old habits. With a major overseas move, a new job, a new city, and a new life, I slowly put about eight pounds back on. I had maintained a lot of my better habits, but my exercise schedule had dropped off quite a bit. So I went back to square one, picked up my bootcamp workbook, and did it all over again. It wasn't as challenging to stay motivated the second time because I already knew it would work as it had for my wedding.

Now, both of us share the cooking responsibilities and made a promise that we would only cook healthy, nutritious meals for each other. Instead of it simply being about my dietary restrictions, it is now about choosing and maintaining a healthy lifestyle for both of us. We do our best to support each other, even though sometimes it would be easier just to order a pizza for delivery.

Today, at seven pounds lighter than I was on my wedding day, I'm feeling great, I have tons of energy, and I'm maintaining my achievement with the support of my husband and the Reserves program.

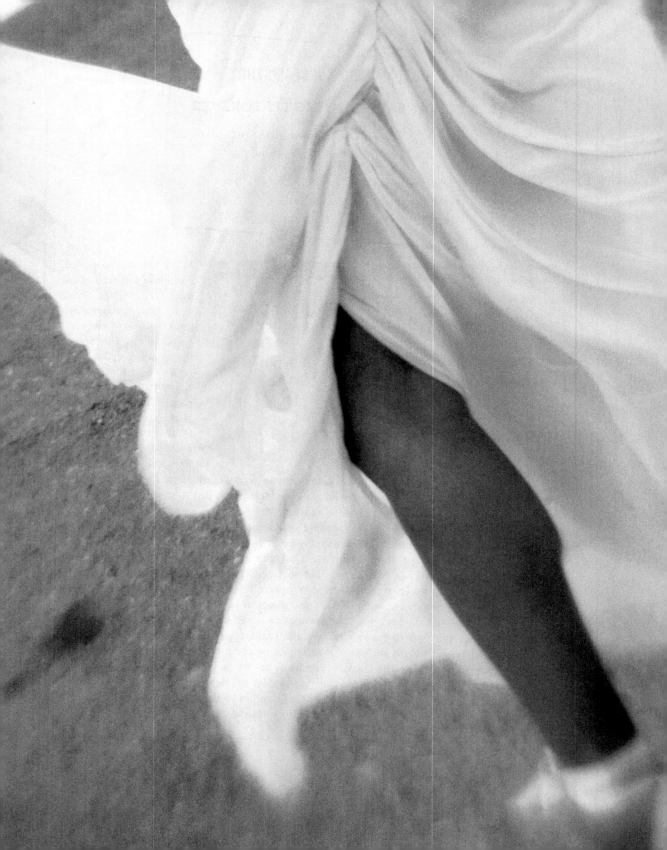

RESERVES

STAYING FIT FOREVER

Welcome back, reservist!

You've been operating in overdrive for months, consumed by the big and small details of your wedding. As you unpack your honeymoon luggage, drop off the film, and settle in to your new life as a married couple, think about your future together and all the wonderful occasions to come.

Now that all the chaos of the wedding is over, you are probably wondering how to turn your weight-loss journey into a lifestyle change. I mentioned earlier that being fit is easier than being fat. And now that you're fit, it makes much more sense to maintain your fabulous new look than to gain the weight back and start all over again. The key is to maintain the exercise routine and healthy eating habits you have developed over the past several months.

Continue to implement the nutritional, motivational, and even accountability "I do's" outlined on pages 19, 23, and 183, exercise regularly, and continue to work toward new goals. Continue to challenge your body by increasing aerobic intensity, always striving for that 6 to 8 aerobic range, and maintain your strength and flexibility routines. This is not the time to move backward!

Do what some of my reservists do: create a danger zone. The danger zone is a range of weight five to ten pounds above your ideal weight. When you reach it, it is time to return to what you learned in Bootcamp360.

For example, you walked down the aisle at your ideal weight of 135 pounds. You left for your honeymoon glowing with the excitement of being a newly married woman. While away, you indulged in romantic dinners and leisurely afternoons on the beach, only to find when you returned that you had gained five pounds. If you continue eating as you did on your honeymoon, all of your hard work will be wasted and you will soon be on the other side of the danger zone, heading quickly back toward your former weight. This is where all the knowledge you accumulated through Bootcamp360 pays off.

Just because the initial goal—your wedding—is over doesn't mean that all your motivation has to go out the window.

Motivation can be found anywhere: Find it in the face of your loving husband, in your family and friends, who are so proud of you for losing weight and getting into shape. Find it in your wedding photos: your portrait is proof that Bootcamp360 works. Think about how you will feel about yourself if you let yourself down and undo all that you have achieved. Is there talk of babies in the future? Staying fit for pregnancy is an important goal. Keep that in mind as you settle into your new life as a married woman.

Find other, small goals that can motivate you. Do you have a party coming up? Is there a charity 10K in the next few months? Have you been invited to a formal party that requires a new cocktail dress? If you look at your schedule, I'm sure you can add a few of your own to the list. You can find a lifetime of goals to work toward. Look at the list below for some ideas. I am sure you can think of a few of your own.

Birthday party in a few weeks
5K for charity next month
A romantic night in with your husband
Holiday party
Beach vacation
New outfit
Girls' night out
Work function
Family reunion
Outdoor activity (skiing or snowboarding)
New fall or spring fashion
Shopping
Other _____

_____

_____

Continue to Increase Your Daily Activity

As you may know, the second part of staying fit and healthy is getting more exercise into your daily routine beyond your hour at the gym. The changes in your daily routine—walking to work instead of driving, getting up to chat with a coworker instead of sending an e-mail—should be second nature now. Every little bit of energy expenditure counts. In fact, research has shown that if you get in twenty minutes of activities daily, you can expend an extra three hundred to four hundred calories a day. This doesn't mean five minutes of high-intensity jumping rope. I am talking about simple daily activities. Review the list below and circle the ones that you can implement. Again, add any to the list that you can think of that may fit your lifestyle.

Vigorous housecleaning
Walking the dog
Walking up the stairs
Standing up while talking on the phone
Parking far away from the grocery store
Doing dishes by hand
Walking to work
Carrying groceries
Walking to a coworker's office instead of e-mailing
Gardening or yard work
Taking the trash out
Walking to get lunch instead of ordering in
Sitting on an exercise ball instead of the couch while watching TV
Doing lunges during commercials
Taking laundry upstairs one load at a time

Always think about why you got into shape to begin with. Your wedding was a great catalyst for getting fit, and now you have the rest of your life with the man you love. I know my husband will always love me unconditionally, and I'm sure yours will too, but I want to be my best regardless. If you are happy with yourself and feel your best, it shows. When he looks at me, I want my husband to always see the stunning, radiant, beautiful bride he married.

CONGRATULATIONS! You are officially a member of the few, the proud, the fit! Keep up with your exercise routine and healthy eating habits and the "hot" you will always be front and center.

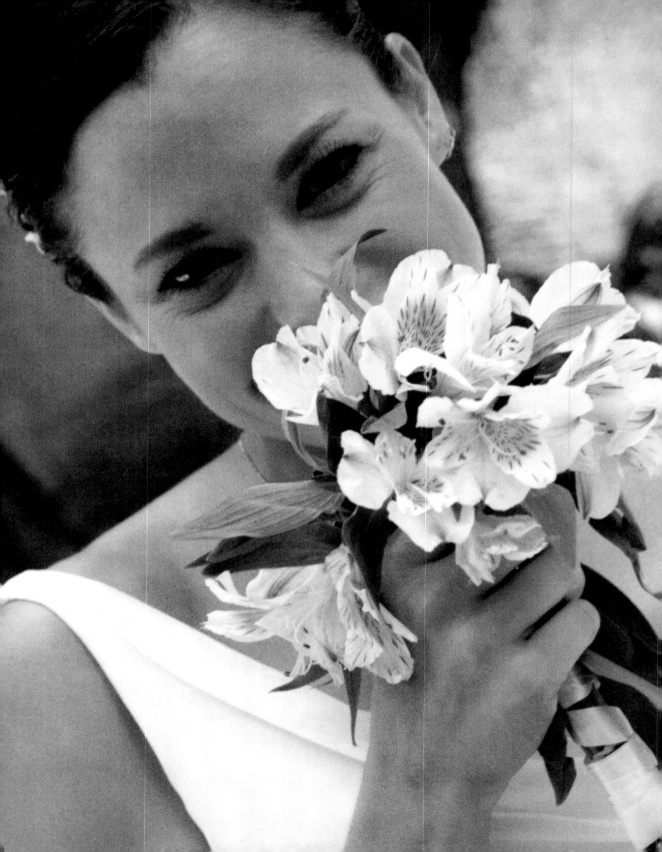

BOOTCAMP360 RESOURCES

No recruit heads into the field without a strategic plan. Sit down in your "war room"—be it your living room, kitchen, or office—and determine your weekly plan of action. What is your plan of attack for exercise and nutrition? When are you going to the gym? What do you need at the grocery store to ensure healthy eating all week? Use these logs to keep you on the straight-and-steady.

APPENDIX A:
PLAN AND PROGRESS LOGS

Track your days. Write down everything you plan to eat and all the exercises you plan to do in the week ahead. Stay accountable to yourself and learn from your actions.

Plan

WEEKLY PLAN	EXERCISE	NUTRITION
Monday	6 a.m.—run around the park—3 miles	Breakfast—egg-white omelet Fruit for snack at work Lunch—salad Dinner—chicken with veggies Lots of water all week!
Tuesday	7 p.m.—Bootcamp Basic at gym	Breakfast—rolled oats with nuts Lunch meeting—order healthy Snacks—bring nutritional bars to work Dinner with fiancé—salmon and broccoli
Wednesday	7 p.m.—kickboxing class at rec center	Breakfast—rolled oats with nuts Lunch—bring lunch today—tuna pita and grilled veggies Dinner—leftovers from last night

Thursday	7 a.m.—Basic in living room
	(have an evening party to go to)
		Breakfast—egg-white omelet
		Lunch with friends—order healthy
		Snacks—bring fruit and edamame to
		   work
		Dinner—steamed veggies and grilled
		   steak salad

Plan (cont'd)

WEEKLY PLAN	EXERCISE	NUTRITION
Friday	10 a.m.—go to gym to lift weights	Breakfast on the go—bring breakfast bar in car Lunch—salad Snacks—bring bars and fruit to work—in car most of the day Dinner with friends—go to fish restaurant
Saturday	10 a.m.—go hiking	Breakfast—egg-white omelet with a piece of turkey bacon Lunch with fiancé—order chicken and veggies Snacks—cut-up veggies for running errands Dinner—eat leftover fish from night before
Sunday	DAY OFF!	DAY OFF! Don't need to record on day off—take a mental and physical break.

Plan and Progress

WEEKLY PLAN	EXERCISE	NUTRITION
Monday		
Tuesday		
Wednesday		
Thursday		
Friday		
Saturday		
Sunday		

APPENDIX B: WEEKLY CHECK-IN LOGS

Once a week, check your weight and track your progress. This will help you make improvements weekly and move toward your monthly goals armed with the knowledge that you are doing all the right things.

The Complete Bootcamp360 Weekly Progress Report

Date: _____

Week #_____

Weight:_____

Size:_____

Fitness:_____

Comments & Thoughts:_____

_____

_____

_____

_____

_____

_____

_____

_____

_____

_____

Note: Measurements are to be done only once a month.

Progress

WEEKLY PLAN	EXERCISE	NUTRITION
Monday	Got up and went running. Felt good about it!	7:30 a.m.—3 egg whites and 1 cup spinach omelet 10 a.m.—orange 1 p.m.—spinach salad with tomatoes and cucumbers, 1 tbs. low-fat ranch dressing 4 p.m.—small bowl of edamame (very hungry) 8 p.m.—1 grilled chicken breast with a plate of veggies and a little olive oil Turned down ice cream. Very proud!
Tuesday	1 hour of Basic, had to go later than planned	7 a.m.—1 cup rolled oats with nuts 10 a.m.—nutritional bar at work 2 p.m.—ordered the fish tacos without rice, extra black beans—no sour cream! Full for the rest of the day 7 p.m.—made salmon and broccoli. Still hungry after, so I ate half a bowl of edamame. Should add some avocado next time.
Wednesday	7 p.m.—kickboxing class. Kicked my butt—felt good!	6 a.m.—rolled oats and nuts Didn't get to snack—in meetings—need to bring more bars to work 1 p.m.—½ pita with tuna and lettuce and a bowl of grilled veggies 4 p.m.—orange 7 p.m.—ate leftovers from last night— 1 serving of salmon and 1 bowl of veggies
Thursday		
Friday		
Saturday		
Sunday		

Progress

WEEKLY PLAN	EXERCISE	NUTRITION
Monday		
Tuesday		
Wednesday		
Thursday		
Friday		
Saturday		
Sunday		

APPENDIX C: EXERCISE LOGS

Every time you perform your strength-training routine, write down the weight used and the repetitions completed. It is imperative that you don't leave this part to guessing. It will help you exercise efficiently while tracking increases in strength.

BASIC		MONDAY		TUESDAY		WEDNESDAY
Warm-up						
Stretch						
Backward Lunge		30 reps		30 reps		30 reps
Plié Squat		30 reps		30 reps		30 reps
Hamstring Roll with Arms Out		30 reps		30 reps		30 reps
Inner-Thigh Ball Squeeze		30 reps		30 reps		30 reps
Outer-Thigh Half-Moon		30 reps		30 reps		30 reps
Standing Calf Raise		30 reps		30 reps		30 reps
Knee Swimmer		30 reps		30 reps		30 reps
Standing Front Raise		30 reps		30 reps		30 reps
One-Arm Exercise Ball Row		30 reps		30 reps		30 reps
Knee Push-up		30 reps		30 reps		30 reps
Chest Press on Exercise Ball		30 reps		30 reps		30 reps
Resistance-Band Pull		30 reps		30 reps		30 reps
Standing Overhead Press with Band		30 reps		30 reps		30 reps
Standing Lateral Raise		30 reps		30 reps		30 reps
Standing Biceps Curl		30 reps		30 reps		30 reps
Hammer Curl with Band		30 reps		30 reps		30 reps

	THURSDAY		FRIDAY		SATURDAY		SUNDAY
	30 reps		30 reps		30 reps		30 reps
	30 reps		30 reps		30 reps		30 reps
	30 reps		30 reps		30 reps		30 reps
	30 reps		30 reps		30 reps		30 reps
	30 reps		30 reps		30 reps		30 reps
	30 reps		30 reps		30 reps		30 reps
	30 reps		30 reps		30 reps		30 reps
	30 reps		30 reps		30 reps		30 reps
	30 reps		30 reps		30 reps		30 reps
	30 reps		30 reps		30 reps		30 reps
	30 reps		30 reps		30 reps		30 reps
	30 reps		30 reps		30 reps		30 reps
	30 reps		30 reps		30 reps		30 reps
	30 reps		30 reps		30 reps		30 reps
	30 reps		30 reps		30 reps		30 reps
	30 reps		30 reps		30 reps		30 reps

BASIC (continued)		MONDAY		TUESDAY		WEDNESDAY
Knee Triceps Push-up		30 reps		30 reps		30 reps
Standing Triceps Press		30 reps		30 reps		30 reps
Exercise Ball Crunch One		30 reps		30 reps		30 reps
Bike on Floor		30 reps		30 reps		30 reps
Dead Bug		30 reps		30 reps		30 reps
Floor Oblique		30 reps		30 reps		30 reps
Exercise Ball Push-Out		30 reps		30 reps		30 reps
Side Toe Touch		30 reps		30 reps		30 reps
Plank		30 seconds		30 seconds		30 seconds
Downward Dog		30 seconds		30 seconds		30 seconds
Spinal Twist		30 seconds		30 seconds		30 seconds
Pigeon		30 seconds		30 seconds		30 seconds
Quadriceps Stretch		30 seconds		30 seconds		30 seconds
Hamstring Stretch		30 seconds		30 seconds		30 seconds
Calf Stretch		30 seconds		30 seconds		30 seconds
Chest and Biceps Stretch		30 seconds		30 seconds		30 seconds
Shoulder Stretch		30 seconds		30 seconds		30 seconds
Triceps Stretch		30 seconds		30 seconds		30 seconds

	THURSDAY		FRIDAY		SATURDAY		SUNDAY
	30 reps		30 reps		30 reps		30 reps
	30 reps		30 reps		30 reps		30 reps
	30 reps		30 reps		30 reps		30 reps
	30 reps		30 reps		30 reps		30 reps
	30 reps		30 reps		30 reps		30 reps
	30 reps		30 reps		30 reps		30 reps
	30 reps		30 reps		30 reps		30 reps
	30 reps		30 reps		30 reps		30 reps
	30 seconds		30 seconds		30 seconds		30 seconds
	30 seconds		30 seconds		30 seconds		30 seconds
	30 seconds		30 seconds		30 seconds		30 seconds
	30 seconds		30 seconds		30 seconds		30 seconds
	30 seconds		30 seconds		30 seconds		30 seconds
	30 seconds		30 seconds		30 seconds		30 seconds
	30 seconds		30 seconds		30 seconds		30 seconds
	30 seconds		30 seconds		30 seconds		30 seconds
	30 seconds		30 seconds		30 seconds		30 seconds
	30 seconds		30 seconds		30 seconds		30 seconds

ADVANCED		MONDAY		TUESDAY		WEDNESDAY
Warm-up						
Stretch						
Backward Lunge with Knee Lift		30 reps		30 reps		30 reps
Plié Squat with Skier Lift		30 reps		30 reps		30 reps
Hamstring Roll on Elbows		30 reps		30 reps		30 reps
Inner-Thigh Exercise Ball Squeeze		30 reps		30 reps		30 reps
Outer-Thigh Half-Moon		30 reps		30 reps		30 reps
Standing Angled Calf Raise		30 reps		30 reps		30 reps
Swimmer on Ball		30 reps		30 reps		30 reps
Seated Front Raise		30 reps		30 reps		30 reps
Bent-Over Row		30 reps		30 reps		30 reps
One-Arm Exercise Ball Chest Press		30 reps		30 reps		30 reps
Straight Push-up off Ball		30 reps		30 reps		30 reps
Standing Overhead Press with Band		30 reps		30 reps		30 reps
Seated Lateral Raise		30 reps		30 reps		30 reps
Seated Biceps Curl		30 reps		30 reps		30 reps
Hammer Curl with Band		30 reps		30 reps		30 reps
Straight Triceps Push-up		30 reps		30 reps		30 reps
Seated Triceps Push-down		30 reps		30 reps		30 reps
Exercise Ball Crunch Two		30 reps		30 reps		30 reps
Bike on Ball		30 reps		30 reps		30 reps
Kayaker		30 reps		30 reps		30 reps

	THURSDAY		FRIDAY		SATURDAY		SUNDAY
	30 reps		30 reps		30 reps		30 reps
	30 reps		30 reps		30 reps		30 reps
	30 reps		30 reps		30 reps		30 reps
	30 reps		30 reps		30 reps		30 reps
	30 reps		30 reps		30 reps		30 reps
	30 reps		30 reps		30 reps		30 reps
	30 reps		30 reps		30 reps		30 reps
	30 reps		30 reps		30 reps		30 reps
	30 reps		30 reps		30 reps		30 reps
	30 reps		30 reps		30 reps		30 reps
	30 reps		30 reps		30 reps		30 reps
	30 reps		30 reps		30 reps		30 reps
	30 reps		30 reps		30 reps		30 reps
	30 reps		30 reps		30 reps		30 reps
	30 reps		30 reps		30 reps		30 reps
	30 reps		30 reps		30 reps		30 reps
	30 reps		30 reps		30 reps		30 reps
	30 reps		30 reps		30 reps		30 reps
	30 reps		30 reps		30 reps		30 reps
	30 reps		30 reps		30 reps		30 reps

ADVANCED (continued)		MONDAY		TUESDAY		WEDNESDAY
Oblique with Leg Lifts		30 reps		30 reps		30 reps
Stick Crunch		30 reps		30 reps		30 reps
Extended Crunch		30 reps		30 reps		30 reps
Ball Balance		30 reps		30 reps		30 reps
Rotating Plank		30 reps		30 reps		30 reps
Downward Dog		30 seconds		30 seconds		30 seconds
Spinal Twist		30 seconds		30 seconds		30 seconds
Pigeon		30 seconds		30 seconds		30 seconds
Quadriceps Stretch		30 seconds		30 seconds		30 seconds
Hamstring Stretch		30 seconds		30 seconds		30 seconds
Calf Stretch		30 seconds		30 seconds		30 seconds
Chest and Biceps Stretch		30 seconds		30 seconds		30 seconds
Shoulder Stretch		30 seconds		30 seconds		30 seconds
Triceps Stretch		30 seconds		30 seconds		30 seconds

	THURSDAY		FRIDAY		SATURDAY		SUNDAY
	30 reps		30 reps		30 reps		30 reps
	30 reps		30 reps		30 reps		30 reps
	30 reps		30 reps		30 reps		30 reps
	30 reps		30 reps		30 reps		30 reps
	30 reps		30 reps		30 reps		30 reps
	30 seconds		30 seconds		30 seconds		30 seconds
	30 seconds		30 seconds		30 seconds		30 seconds
	30 seconds		30 seconds		30 seconds		30 seconds
	30 seconds		30 seconds		30 seconds		30 seconds
	30 seconds		30 seconds		30 seconds		30 seconds
	30 seconds		30 seconds		30 seconds		30 seconds
	30 seconds		30 seconds		30 seconds		30 seconds
	30 seconds		30 seconds		30 seconds		30 seconds
	30 seconds		30 seconds		30 seconds		30 seconds

HARD CORE		MONDAY		TUESDAY		WEDNESDAY
Warm-up						
Stretch						
Backward Lunge with Punches		30 reps		30 reps		30 reps
Squat Kicks		30 reps		30 reps		30 reps
Hamstring Roll, No Arms		30 reps		30 reps		30 reps
Inner-Thigh Lift		30 reps		30 reps		30 reps
Outer-Thigh Half-Moon		30 reps		30 reps		30 reps
Standing Angled Calf Raise		30 reps		30 reps		30 reps
Lift and Rotate		30 reps		30 reps		30 reps
Seated Leg-Lifted Front Raise		30 reps		30 reps		30 reps
Overhead Raise on Ball		30 reps		30 reps		30 reps
Wide Row on Ball		30 reps		30 reps		30 reps
Push-up on Ball		30 reps		30 reps		30 reps
Chest Fly on Ball		30 reps		30 reps		30 reps
Standing Overhead Press with Band		30 reps		30 reps		30 reps
Seated Leg-Lifted Lateral Raise		30 reps		30 reps		30 reps
Seated Leg-Lifted Biceps Curl		30 reps		30 reps		30 reps
Hammer Curl with Band		30 reps		30 reps		30 reps
Triceps Push-down		30 reps		30 reps		30 reps
Triceps Dip off Ball		30 reps		30 reps		30 reps
Kickback on Ball		30 reps		30 reps		30 reps
Exercise Ball Crunch Three		30 reps		30 reps		30 reps
Bike on Ball		30 reps		30 reps		30 reps

THURSDAY		FRIDAY		SATURDAY		SUNDAY
	30 reps		30 reps		30 reps		30 reps
	30 reps		30 reps		30 reps		30 reps
	30 reps		30 reps		30 reps		30 reps
	30 reps		30 reps		30 reps		30 reps
	30 reps		30 reps		30 reps		30 reps
	30 reps		30 reps		30 reps		30 reps
	30 reps		30 reps		30 reps		30 reps
	30 reps		30 reps		30 reps		30 reps
	30 reps		30 reps		30 reps		30 reps
	30 reps		30 reps		30 reps		30 reps
	30 reps		30 reps		30 reps		30 reps
	30 reps		30 reps		30 reps		30 reps
	30 reps		30 reps		30 reps		30 reps
	30 reps		30 reps		30 reps		30 reps
	30 reps		30 reps		30 reps		30 reps
	30 reps		30 reps		30 reps		30 reps
	30 reps		30 reps		30 reps		30 reps
	30 reps		30 reps		30 reps		30 reps
	30 reps		30 reps		30 reps		30 reps
	30 reps		30 reps		30 reps		30 reps
	30 reps		30 reps		30 reps		30 reps

HARD CORE (CONTINUED)		MONDAY		TUESDAY		WEDNESDAY
Oblique on Ball		30 reps		30 reps		30 reps
Rolling Jackknife		30 reps		30 reps		30 reps
Kayaker with Legs		30 reps		30 reps		30 reps
Rotating Plank		30 seconds		30 seconds		30 seconds
Downward Dog		30 seconds		30 seconds		30 seconds
Spinal Twist		30 seconds		30 seconds		30 seconds
Pigeon		30 seconds		30 seconds		30 seconds
Quadriceps Stretch		30 seconds		30 seconds		30 seconds
Hamstring Stretch		30 seconds		30 seconds		30 seconds
Calf Stretch		30 seconds		30 seconds		30 seconds
Chest and Biceps Stretch		30 seconds		30 seconds		30 seconds
Shoulder Stretch		30 seconds		30 seconds		30 seconds
Triceps Stretch		30 seconds		30 seconds		30 seconds

THURSDAY		FRIDAY		SATURDAY		SUNDAY
30 reps		30 reps		30 reps		30 reps
30 reps		30 reps		30 reps		30 reps
30 reps		30 reps		30 reps		30 reps
30 seconds		30 seconds		30 seconds		30 seconds
30 seconds		30 seconds		30 seconds		30 seconds
30 seconds		30 seconds		30 seconds		30 seconds
30 seconds		30 seconds		30 seconds		30 seconds
30 seconds		30 seconds		30 seconds		30 seconds
30 seconds		30 seconds		30 seconds		30 seconds
30 seconds		30 seconds		30 seconds		30 seconds
30 seconds		30 seconds		30 seconds		30 seconds
30 seconds		30 seconds		30 seconds		30 seconds
30 seconds		30 seconds		30 seconds		30 seconds

WEDDING WEEK		MONDAY		TUESDAY		WEDNESDAY
Jumping jacks		50 reps		50 reps		50 reps
Squats		20 reps		20 reps		20 reps
Lunges, each leg		20 reps		20 reps		20 reps
Stretch		1 min.		1 min.		1 min.
Squats—Vary tempo		5 min.		5 min.		5 min.
Jump rope		1 min.		1 min.		1 min.
Chest—Vary tempo		5 min.		5 min.		5 min.
Run in place		1 min.		1 min.		1 min.
Triceps—Vary tempo		5 min.		5 min.		5 min.
Jump rope		1 min.		1 min.		1 min.
Lunges—Vary tempo		5 min.		5 min.		5 min.
Jumping jacks		1 min.		1 min.		1 min.
Back—Vary tempo		5 min.		5 min.		5 min.
Squat 180		1 min.		1 min.		1 min.
Biceps—Vary tempo		5 min.		5 min.		5 min.
Jumping jacks		1 min.		1 min.		1 min.
Shoulders—Vary tempo		5 min.		5 min.		5 min.
Abs/lower back		10 min.		10 min.		10 min.
Stretch/cool down		5 min.		5 min.		5 min.

THURSDAY		FRIDAY		SATURDAY		SUNDAY
50 reps		50 reps		50 reps		50 reps
20 reps		20 reps		20 reps		20 reps
20 reps		20 reps		20 reps		20 reps
1 min.		1 min.		1 min.		1 min.
5 min.		5 min.		5 min.		5 min.
1 min.		1 min.		1 min.		1 min.
5 min.		5 min.		5 min.		5 min.
1 min.		1 min.		1 min.		1 min.
5 min.		5 min.		5 min.		5 min.
1 min.		1 min.		1 min.		1 min.
5 min.		5 min.		5 min.		5 min.
1 min.		1 min.		1 min.		1 min.
5 min.		5 min.		5 min.		5 min.
1 min.		1 min.		1 min.		1 min.
5 min.		5 min.		5 min.		5 min.
1 min.		1 min.		1 min.		1 min.
5 min.		5 min.		5 min.		5 min.
10 min.		10 min.		10 min.		10 min.
5 min.		5 min.		5 min.		5 min.

INDEX